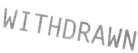

Chasing Hope

blue
rider
press

ALSO BY RICHARD M. COHEN

Blindsided

Strong at the Broken Places

I Want to Kill the Dog

Chasing Hope

A Patient's Deep Dive into
Stem Cells, Faith, and the Future

Richard M. Cohen

BLUE RIDER PRESS

New York

blue
rider
press

An imprint of Penguin Random House LLC
375 Hudson Street
New York, New York 10014

Blue Rider Press is a registered trademark and its colophon
is a trademark of Penguin Random House LLC

ISBN 9780399575259 (hardcover)
ISBN 9780399575273 (ebook)

Printed in the United States of America
1   3   5   7   9   10   8   6   4   2

Book design by Amy Hill

For Mimi and Grandpa, my late parents,
who offered unqualified love
to four generations
and never lost hope

Hope is easy for the foolish, but hard for the wise.
Everybody can lose himself into foolish hope,
but genuine hope is something rare and great.

—PAUL TILLICH

CONTENTS

CONTENTS

PREFACE

I don't like prefaces and rarely read them. When I care enough to put my hands on a good book, I just want to get started. Frequently there is ground to cover before a reader turns a page. I get it. So here is my reluctant preface. Be assured it is short. Really short. Please forgive the statistics, but the numbers speak loudly about our need for hope.

According to the Centers for Disease Control, more than 117 million Americans live with at least one chronic condition. That is almost half the population of the United States. Chronic illnesses were responsible for seven of the ten leading causes of death in 2010. This is serious stuff. To add to that, almost 20 percent of us are disabled. We are a people in need.

Chronic conditions are incurable and can play out over a lifetime. They become more common as we age, and we are fast becoming the oldest population in American history. Chronic illnesses include heart disease, diabetes and obesity, some cancers, and numerous neurological disorders. The list is long. I am disabled and grapple with a few of these dread diseases myself. Lucky me.

Multiple sclerosis rules my life. Fading vision and limbs that no longer function properly, cognitive issues, and dizzying imbalance have become my new normal. I am a different person than the one I used to know. Each day is a challenge to be met and mastered. But I am grateful for what I have.

The struggle against illness has been going on through the ages. Women and men of the world have longed to know hope since time immemorial. That never has been more true than today. In America, we live under a state of siege from an army of illnesses. Americans seem to believe this is more about the other guy than the person we see in the mirror. But most of us will be touched by serious sickness in our lifetimes. Sooner or later we cross paths with hope. For many, that is all we have

Our sons and daughters, spouses and siblings, friends and neighbors, our colleagues and the cops on the corner may have a problem or two we do not see. We do not know who is next in line. That is a mystery of life. I believe life is an exploration. My journey into the land of hope took me to new places. In many ways, I began the investigation in 2012, when an invitation to a stem cell conference at the Vatican caused me to reevaluate the last decade of my, and my family's, relationship with hope, faith, and the future.

Throughout the next five years, first as a journalist, then as a blogger, I explored hope in its many forms. I visited families touched by serious illnesses and interviewed religious leaders. I attended Friday prayers with immigrant Muslims and participated in that stem cell conference, which led me to an experimental treatment for MS.

I covered a lot of ground and learned as much about myself and my relationship to hope as I did about the treatment itself. I am a person for whom hope does not come easy. The journey was worthwhile. Ultimately, I decided to accept intelligent risk and cast my fate to the wind. I realize there are many views of hope, and all of us must find our own and embrace it.

Now, please read.

Chasing Hope

CHAPTER 1

Losing Sight of the Future

O n a dark, blustery afternoon in the autumn of 2010, I joined a ragtag army of New York City commuters waiting to board a bus that would lumber downtown. Heavy rain pelted everyone in line. We were stepping over puddles and negotiating the steep, slippery stairs, trying not to break a leg or let ourselves be blown away.

As I slid into one of the last remaining seats, the bus started up again and began slowly making its way down Broadway, the Great White Way I knew so well. I would be disembarking before we hit the theater district, as I had done a thousand times. I glanced out the fogged window to see the stores and restaurants that had long served as my landmarks.

I was numb, less from the chill than from the fact that in recent days it had become clear that after years of relatively stable sight, I was losing yet more vision due to complications from multiple sclerosis. MS is my constant companion. It is

1

an incurable inflammatory, degenerative, progressive, auto-immune chronic illness. Whatever. Not only is my vision flee-ing, but my lateral judgment is also compromised, which accounts for the bruises on my arms and legs from bumping into furniture and glancing off doorways. Sometimes I felt I needed football pads just to walk the streets of New York.

The bus was headed to where I wanted to go, the MS was not, though both were going south. The disease was active, dancing through much of my body. The neurological predator was focusing once again on my eyes. If I lost any more sight, I feared I would lose my ability to function as a writer, not to mention as a husband and father.

Suddenly I sat up ramrod straight as I realized I had no idea where I was. I could not make out the storefronts outside the window. They were lost in a foggy blur, fading to vague shapes and drab colors. Buildings were melting into unrecog-nizable blobs. I felt as if I had been kidnapped and was being transported to an alien place. I froze. My reflexive denial, usu-ally a well-oiled machine, stalled out. Frantically, I attempted to peer through the fog, trying to identify anything that would tell me my location. I just could not make that happen. I turned my attention to the driver. He was yelling at an el-derly woman, telling her where to get off the bus. That was what I needed to hear. I listened and figured out our current location then counted the stops until I knew it was time to struggle down the stairs.

I emerged into a strange city that I could barely make out. Nothing looked right. Sights and sounds were exaggerated. Cars seemed to move at double speed. *Please don't do this*, I silently cried out. *Don't let me lose my sight.* I was pleading with nobody; I had long ago given up on the idea of a deity coming to the rescue. That narrowed my options.

This kind of panic was unknown to me. During my years as a producer at CBS News, I had worked alongside type A personalities who drank coffee so strong you could eat it with a fork, people who constantly hyperventilated their way around the office. I was not one of them. I was labeled a type Z personality. It's only television, I used to say. Not worth making yourself crazy.

Anxiety gripped me so hard that now *I* was the one hyperventilating. As I stood struggling to see the other side of a busy avenue, I was in full emotional retreat. I wanted to cry. Usually, I am a guy with a penchant for gallows humor. Now I could not find my reservoir of old, bad jokes.

I had been legally blind for some time. This was something different. I knew a crisis when I saw one. There I was, standing in a cold rain on a busy street corner and wondering where to turn for help.

I managed to get my bearings. My friend Charlie Osgood's apartment was right across the street. Praise be. Charlie is as calming in person as he is on television, and he helped me get emotionally righted. My anxiety level was reduced, but not by much. There was work to do. The first step was to see if I could reel in my missing vision.

T he next day, I was in safe territory. I made my way to the infusion suite at the Tisch MS Research Center. The office was dry and warm and strangely welcoming. I had performed this medical ritual many times when alarm bells sounded. But the voices around me were comforting because I knew the people they belonged to, not because they were in possession of a magic bullet.

Out came the Solu-Medrol, the old steroid warrior, an all-purpose drug used to treat conditions as varied as arthritis, disorders of the blood and the immune system, severe allergic responses, certain cancers, eye conditions, and skin, kidney, intestinal, and lung diseases. One size fits all.

I have been getting infusions of this stuff for years, mostly for lack of a more effective elixir. It fights inflammation, a contributing problem with MS, but it offers no promise of long-term change, only short-term relief. Often not even that. I would have preferred a martini.

As the steroid flowed into a vein in my arm, it left the usual metallic taste in my mouth. I sat and stared at nothing in particular, wondering if any part of my missing sight would reappear. Days after the infusion, the immediate crisis might end. It might not. You put your money down and take your chances. I would have to wait a few weeks to see if my condition stabilized or even improved. Based on my history, it was unlikely it would get much better. The drug has never carried me back to the starting line. But for no extra charge, the poison does bring on madness and violent mood swings to go with certain serious sleep deprivation. I knew I would be a mess, but when vision has been lost, you do what you have to and hope there will be a payoff.

Maybe my missing vision would crawl at least halfway home this time. I would settle for that. I am used to settling. In the MS world, patients make do with what we can get. By now I understand that I always am waiting for Godot. I am tired of being dragged to the theater when I am pretty sure I know how the play ends.

A few weeks after the infusion, a portion of my diminished vision did grudgingly return. With the small improvement came the need for a midcourse correction. There would be new lenses, adjusted expectations, an even greater tolerance for ambiguity required. Not knowing if the improvement will last has become a way of life for me.

In my well-worn speech to myself, I advised only that I keep my middle finger pointed north. That would keep the piss and vinegar circulating and serve as my compass. If that is self-indulgent, so be it. Anger can be its own command to keep fighting.

Once I learned I had MS, I watched my father closely for clues of what would happen to me. My Old Man died at ninety, having lived with MS for seventy years. The truth is that after my dad retired, he had many good years and seemed strong until he reached his eighties. It was only in the last decade of his life that he withdrew, effectively shutting himself off. Once a hearty traveler, he stopped doing much and had to be coaxed out of the house. In his final years, he was in a motorized wheelchair. The Old Man seemed to surrender to a reality he knew he could not alter.

I did not inherit his common sense or the willingness to recognize when it was time to raise the white flag. But my symptoms have become severe at a much younger age than his did. I already recognize my periods of withdrawing, as he had done in his old age, shutting people out during tough times. "Get out of your head," a shrink once advised me. "Engage with others."

I do not much like myself as the solitary soldier, but sometimes I cannot help retreating into my head. It seems to be the only safe place where I can hide. I spend considerable time there. The entrance to my cave is firmly closed, secured with a lock only I can open. Even my close friends are kept at arm's length.

My wife, Meredith, warns me not to shut myself away and become my father. I tell Meredith not to become my mother, who was fiercely loyal to the Old Man and stayed by his side to the end, joining him in forfeiting freedom. I don't believe Meredith will sacrifice her own life to my illness. Her life is too full for that. I am not so sure about myself. My anger and frustration sometimes are overwhelming.

Hope can be an antidote to situational anger. Sometimes the two are served at the same table, one from column A, the other column B. Be warned. Anger and hope are improbable plate mates. They are never served in equal proportions or at the same temperatures. They do not mix well. Anger can be quite spicy; hope, bland. Anger is a mean mixture, bitter to the taste, toxic to the system. Maybe hope is a glass of warm milk; drink it before bed and sleep well. I seem more temperamentally inclined toward anger.

I kept reminding myself that I am more than my illness. Who I am is in my head and heart, in my soul, not in my sneakers. I had to find a way to rise above the daily grind of illness. That is a test of faith in the future. Perhaps it is a fancy synonym for *hope*. Whatever it is, I was having a hard time doing it.

CHAPTER 2

The Diagnosis

Back in 1973, my immune system declared war on my body. I became aware of troubling neurological impulses, signals that something was wrong. I was living in Washington, D.C., where I had moved to work on Capitol Hill. I fell into journalism, working for *Issues and Answers*, the old ABC News Sunday public affairs program. Upward mobility was easy for me then. I became an associate producer and worked with Frank Reynolds and Ted Koppel. Life was good.

I never tired of walking to work, cutting through the Capitol and down the hill to the ABC News bureau. I would amble past the White House and smile at the demonstrators who were always there. Each morning I shook hands with a man carrying a sign announcing that the CIA had implanted electrodes in his brain. I was happy to call myself a journalist.

Back in 1973, I left ABC for PBS, where I helped produce a program in a series called *America '73*, hosted by Robin

MacNeil and Jim Lehrer. My hour was on the politics of disability in America. As we were editing the film, I realized I was having strange sensations. I fell a few times but ignored it. One leg felt numb, which I assumed was a psychological reaction to spending time with contemporaries sitting in wheelchairs.

My dad called one evening, mostly to gossip about President Nixon, who was mired in the Watergate scandal. I told him about my symptoms, and he urged me to see a doctor. We chatted briefly and hung up.

Minutes later, my dad called again. "I think you have multiple sclerosis," he calmly told me. The Old Man knew the drill. Not only was he a physician, but he had been living with multiple sclerosis himself for many decades. My grandmother, my dad's mother, had MS too. It appeared that the disease might be a family heirloom, passed down to another generation.

I knew surprisingly little about the illness, given that someone so close to me suffered from it. My parents were products of a culture that valued silence on issues of personal health. My father's ups and downs had become closely held secrets, and I was oblivious to his struggles. I had no basis for processing what a life with multiple sclerosis would mean.

As the son and grandson of people battling the disease, maybe I should have seen this possible diagnosis coming. But nothing I had read or heard suggested there was a genetic link. I was just living my life, assuming I was Superman, like all strapping twenty-five-year-old men do. I was covering the Watergate hearings, witnessing history. I had no time for neurological nonsense.

I did eventually see a neurologist on a spring day in 1973. The doctor conducted a thorough exam and ordered a spinal tap to determine if there was protein in my spinal fluid, one of the indicators of MS. There was. I had a roaring spinal headache and no peace of mind.

The official diagnosis came a few days later. It was bad news. My life sentence was delivered in a quick phone call. The neurologist must have figured the headline did not warrant a face-to-face meeting. That doctor had the people skills of a prison guard, minus the charm.

The ground beneath my feet had shifted. Never again would I be the guy I had always seen in the mirror. The doctor had bluntly made clear there was little he could do, code for "nothing at all." I could have used some encouragement, some hope, but none was offered. It was diagnose and adios, as the saying went.

After the phone call, I sat in an old chair in my third-floor walk-up on Capitol Hill. I silently stared until twilight took over outside the windows. I began scanning my tired, shabby apartment. There was nothing in the room but torn wallpaper and a worn couch. Suddenly it struck me that I was in worse shape than the furniture.

I wanted to distance myself from the news. I surprised

myself by making a few quick decisions. The first was not to freak out. Perhaps the decision not to lose it was a sign of nascent hope, that remaining calm could have a palliative effect on my emotions.

I knew what I did not know about MS, which was almost everything. I could not even spell *multiple sclerosis*. And now I knew that MS was my new life sentence.

I scoured my memory for details about how my grandmother and my father fought the disease. My grandmother, Celia, was a strong, eccentric woman whose struggles with MS were largely invisible to me until late in her life. Celia sat in a wheelchair but could break an apple in half cleanly, twisting it between her bare hands. How sick could she have been? Celia was never officially diagnosed with the illness, though it now seems clear that it was MS that had left her in a permanent sitting position. This was decades before imaging, and the tests were endless and often unpleasant. The diagnostic process was difficult in those days. No one wanted to put her through that ordeal, especially since there were no treatments back then.

I did not even know my father was sick until I was in my first year of college, barely six years before my own diagnosis. He called a family press conference one day, made the announcement, and took no questions. I felt as if Nixon had just left the room. My dad had seemed to be doing well, but no one except my mother really knew. And she was not talking.

My dad had been diagnosed when he was twenty years

old, during his first year of medical school. He temporarily lost vision in one eye. Later he developed double vision. That did not stop him from finishing medical school when he was twenty-four. He became an anesthesiologist, then a pediatric anesthesiologist, putting young kids under and keeping them alive during surgery. To me, that line of work was unimaginable, but he could do it because he kept his cool. That served him well when dealing with his own illness. He continued working until he was sixty-three, when he could no longer wheel the young patients back to their rooms after surgery.

The Old Man wore his illness well, and he never lost his sense of humor. He lived a full life and was a role model for me. His resolve was contagious. So was his realism. When I wrote *Blindsided*, my memoir, I asked my father if he would mind if I called him the Old Man. "I would expect nothing less" was his answer.

My doctor's implicit message, which I had received loud and clear, was that there was no hope. I never had thought about that word in the context of my health. For me, hope was about winning promotions or getting a date, not staying healthy and alive. And now I had been told to forget about help or hope. This was a devastating message to give to a young man of twenty-five.

I rebounded quickly. Or rather, I went into deep denial. I was athletic and ambitious, and because I was for the most part without symptoms, I looked and felt healthy. So I decided to just ignore my diagnosis and assume that I would remain well. I was being defiant rather than realistic, but I had accidently discovered a coping mechanism that served me well for years.

So began the long and uncertain process of redefining myself. I assumed I had to shape a new plan for my future. What that meant was unclear. Everything seemed to defy explanation, but I was confident that I could take care of myself. This was pure bravado on my part, but I felt I had to act it out, even on shaky legs.

There can be no doubt that determination is embedded in my DNA. Just like the Old Man had, I decided this sickness would remain under wraps. I would keep quiet, and I would prevail. The Old Man lived with a secret sickness and urged me to do the same. I never heard him complain, and I was careful never to complain in front of him. The one time he heard me ask, "Why me?" he responded quickly, calling me a professional asshole. I did not make that mistake again.

Determination and denial carried me far, though I struggled with knowing how much denial was too much. MS was breaking down my door. Eventually, the disease was no longer a stranger, but it still treated me with cold dispatch. I began to feel truly disabled. Physical abilities fell away like dry leaves. I thought of the days when my wife, Meredith, and I used to hike together, climbing the steep ski slopes of summer and breathing free. In the fall, we would bike back roads as the foliage changed, turning green to gold. Soon enough, I knew biking was in my rearview mirror.

Over the years, I kept moving as best as I could, even though I had to walk with my eyes pointed down, stepping carefully, since I could trip over obstacles as tiny as sidewalk cracks. One would have thought I was on the lookout for loose change. I have been on the streets of Paris and hardly noticed the Eiffel Tower for fear of tripping over a cobblestone.

Those of us who grapple each day with physical flaws must program ourselves to take the safe, paved path to get us where we are headed. In due time, we reach our destinations. Taking the well-traveled road can be boring, but it gets me there.

A life of being without doing is boring, and boredom is among life's fiercest foes. The safe, sedentary existence is not for me. My years of being an adventure addict and living dangerously around the world for better or worse made me who I am. Now Meredith gets on my case for jaywalking. How the mighty have fallen. But crossing a busy avenue against a green light is about as much adventure as I am able to enjoy. That is not a recipe for longevity, especially being legally blind, but it will have to do. Risk for its own sake is foolish. I know that.

Serious sickness too frequently defines a life. We become whatever condition afflicts us. How we believe others see us can be a powerful force. Who we see in the mirror each morning defines our sense of self. We fall back on personal strength and the power of a loving family.

CHAPTER 3

Meredith and Company

During my early years on the *CBS Evening News*, I crossed paths with a Chicago-based correspondent named Meredith Vieira. It was contempt at first sight, as we both like to say. We tentatively circled each other, two-legged animals stalking their prey.

I once found Meredith lying on a couch in her office, watching *Looney Tunes*. I immediately trashed her. Sarcasm is a wonderful mechanism for flirting. Meredith later wandered into my editing room and screened a story I was cutting. She ridiculed it. That exchange gave birth to a dynamic still in play: giving each other a hard time and cutting no slack.

Meredith and I married in 1986. I had told her about the MS in the earliest days of our relationship because I wanted us to deal with the subject before we got too serious. She never flinched. We hiked and biked, traveled and jogged, wherever we went. We owned the world.

Both of us knew we wanted a family. Genetic counseling was in its infancy, and we gave little thought to the possibility of passing along the illness. There were four miscarriages, but we kept trying. Ben was born in 1989. A few years later, along came Gabe, and soon after our daughter, Lily, showed up. Life had been good. Now it was great.

The changes in my body came gradually and were subtle enough that only I knew about them. There was diminished function in my arms and legs. Bouts of MS-related optic neuritis, the condition that had caused the dimming of both eyes in the early stages of the disease, kept striking in the night.

I was on a slow slide down, but I still believed I could reverse direction. I was not going to allow deteriorating health and vision to rob me of my faith in myself. This was not a hope. In my mind, it was a certainty. I was adept at appearing to be strong. Looking and sounding sturdy allowed me to believe I *was* strong. In retrospect, this was wishful thinking, but it worked. My strongman persona served its purpose, even though I had been inching toward legal blindness since finishing my degree at Columbia. Progressive diseases progress, however, and MS chips away at a body, and eventually the swaggering television news producer had to be phased out of his own movie. Reluctantly, in the late 1990s, I realized I had to leave the business.

I missed the person I used to be. Producers are tough individuals who jump out of airplanes without parachutes, land on their feet in strange lands, and get the job done. That was no longer possible. In my own eyes, I was a diminished man. I was going to have to reinvent myself. For a while I consulted for foundations and other nonprofits, work I found too slow for one accustomed to demanding deadlines.

Our kids were young and revved up to absorb every bit of attention they could get from their parents. I increased my involvement in their lives. I quickly realized that should have been happening under any circumstances. Our children sucked up the attention. I loved it. Men frequently bury themselves in their jobs, too often oblivious to what they are failing to give to their families. I look back and see this as a good time in my life.

My three kids knew I was sick as they grew up, though no scary-sounding name for my condition was attached for a long time. Their first moment of concern for their father probably came one evening when they still were in elementary school. They were gathered on the second floor as I climbed the stairs on my way to wish them good night. On the way up, a leg gave out and down I went, headfirst and backward.

I had not performed this trick for an audience before. They did not visibly react, but the show certainly had an effect on them. Later, Meredith sat with Ben when the lights were out and he was tucked into bed. In our house, that was when our kids talked most freely.

"Mom," Ben began. "Is what is wrong with Dad what Grandpa has?" Meredith fudged her answer and made her way into our bedroom, where she let me know that she felt the time had come to talk to the kids and put a name on my neurological nemesis. I do not remember a lot about my conversation with Ben, except that I tried not to sugarcoat the situation.

We had learned the hard way that if you want happy, secure kids, tell them the truth. They are the smartest creatures in the house. Kids talk to one another. Their ears pick up every word they overhear. Children just seem to absorb family news.

Not long after, life under our roof changed. And I changed. My self-esteem was suffering. I felt like my weakness was out there for all the world to see. Others had no clue about what was going on in my head, but the ground under my feet had shifted.

Then came the earthquake that upended our lives. I often relive the horrible moment on a train platform one afternoon almost twenty-five years ago. The horror is as fresh as if the accident had occurred yesterday.

In 1992, I accidentally knocked Ben down into the small space between a commuter train and the platform. *The New York Times Magazine* column About Men published my account of the event. As we stepped off the train, "he tumbled into that narrow space like a shiny penny disappearing into a piggy bank. It was a slow-motion movie sequence, and I was powerless to stop it. A quick glance up at me, devoid of all expression, and he vanished. Our careful choreography of parent watching over child had gone awry. The grown-up caution that guides the movements of a little boy, not yet 4, had broken down. Failed."

Ben and I had boarded the train for a ride up the river. Once we were on the train, I looked back and saw my CNN ID lying on the platform, where I must have dropped it. I told Ben to stay in the car and stepped off the train to fetch it. My failing vision did not track Ben following me. I lost my balance and lurched backward, knocking my son into the space between the train and platform.

"I froze for an instant and realized I had to act fast. I pleaded with startled travelers not to let the doors close. Trains with open doors don't move. People were horrified and motionless. Mannequins. I guess no one knew what to do. My God, I quickly wondered, where is the third rail humming with electricity? The toaster with a knife sticking out."

A group of passengers blocked the closing doors. I fell to my knees, leaning into the space and trying not to slip and get wedged in. I yelled for Ben to reach up toward my voice. I panicked, fearing I would not find his arms. But we locked hands, and Ben was returned to the platform.

Ben survived with barely a scratch, but I was damaged for many years, afraid to be alone while guarding my kids. I had failed and was not confident that if given a second chance I would be so lucky again. Ben thought he remembered the incident because he heard the story repeated so often by family and friends. I kept busy trying to purge my mind.

I still have flashes of terror that run through me like a bolt of lightning. To this day, I look at my grown children and wonder how they survived me.

Any parent knows that eyes cannot wander away from youngsters, even for a moment. Yet I was learning that vigilance cannot always compensate for physical flaws. So I began to overcompensate. In the subway, one part of my kids' bodies had to be touching the wall. The kids thought that was goofy, but it was the law of the land when Dad was in charge. Period. Future adventures depended on compliance now, but our outings were still fun. No one could tell that my heart was spending time in my throat. It took years to shake that vulnerable feeling. As they moved quickly, I lagged behind. My walking was slowing. When we went out together, they arrived at every street corner before I could catch up. They knew not to cross without me, but I feared memory would fail if they saw a friend or even a dog across the street.

As the kids' ages approached double digits, my physical condition worsened. After decades of getting off easy with my body, the MS was catching up with me. Finally, I had to wear my disability openly. I had no choice. I worried my kids would see me as I saw myself: damaged. I feared they would feel they had been robbed of the dad they all wanted, a father able to walk in their world. I never saw a sign of that, but I still felt deprived of the opportunity to be a normal father.

Ben and Gabe became aspiring athletes as they approached adolescence. Our lives suddenly included soccer and baseball, cross-country and golf, any sport they considered competitive. I had hoped to throw baseballs and footballs with the boys, to play touch football in neighborhood pickup games.

Keeping up with Ben and Gabe was a struggle for me, but they seemed not to notice. The boys turned every activity into a blood sport. I could stop worrying about killing them. They were well on their way to killing each other. Lily seemed to view them as martians and focused on her acting.

The kids and I invented our own games. The boys didn't appear to be fazed by my limitations. Instead, those difficulties were built into the games we created. There was baseball, with one player unable to see well enough to catch a ball. I did not even try hitting. I threw the best line drives and deep fly balls I could, and the boys competed with each other to reach the ball first. We created driveway hockey, slapping around a tennis ball with old hockey sticks. The contest featured Pierre WaWa, a broken-down veteran player with weak legs and a bad limp. Ben played hard, cutting me no slack. I liked that. All along, the issues were not with my arms and legs but in my head. These kids loved playing with Dad. That was all that mattered to them. It took a while for me to recognize that.

My hopes for more perfect arms and legs receded, and my

condition kept worsening. I was losing the ability to do much of anything that was physically rigorous, so we moved indoors and hung out at a chessboard. Ben often beat me and was stunned whenever he heard me utter "checkmate."

The boys continued to grow up, and they left me in the dust. Dad was traded to the minors as their athletic skills sharpened and they joined school teams. I was in the stands at every game and never missed a play Lily was in, though I barely could see the stage. I loved being a dad.

Meredith and I worked in news, a hypercompetitive world. There are neither medals nor merit badges for staying home with the kids. We did it, and it was great. Our children clearly have a deep comfort level with us. Meredith and I had an agreement that we would not travel on business at the same time. One of us would always be home. Our mantra and vow to ourselves was simple. Be there.

CHAPTER 4

An Unwanted Inheritance

MS has a genetic component, but neither my parents nor Meredith and I understood that when we decided to have children. I had become aware of familial connections through the years, punctuated by my own diagnosis with MS. Complicated emotions find their way to the surface when I worry about MS hitting my children.

The nightmare scenario does not go away. I feel powerless before my fears. Meredith is right there with me and worries as much as I do. Still, I am alone with my worst fears. That issue was in its usual spot in the back of my mind when I came across an online column in *The Washington Post*'s Health and Science section in late 2016. My inquiry into hope was just under way, and the prospect of reading about a father passing along a disease to a son was horrifying.

The headline stopped me cold: "'My Heart Breaks 80

Million Ways': A Father Passes a Disorder to His Son." The author, Carl Luepker, was a forty-four-year-old former sixth-grade math teacher in Minneapolis, who described his long battle with dystonia.

Dystonia is a debilitating neurological condition, causing the muscles of the body to contract involuntarily, which results in repetitive or twisting movements. These movements can interfere with the performance of many day-to-day tasks, even some as basic as the ability to use a pen or pencil. Join the club, I thought.

Dystonia generally begins in either the hands or the feet and gradually progresses to the rest of the body. The disease can eventually affect the ability to speak. The psychological impact can be devastating when only a speaker understands what he or she is saying.

When Carl and his wife, Heather, a speech-language pathologist, thought about starting a family, they considered the risks of passing his illness on to another generation. They decided to roll the dice, he told me. "If I did carry the gene, there would be a one-in-six chance that our kid would develop the disorder. Heather said, 'Well, then you'll have to coach them through it. We will love them regardless.'"

Their son, Liam, did develop the disease. Their daughter, Lucia, did not. Carl wrote in the *Post* of how hard it is for him to see his child suffering. "I can live with my bad luck in getting this condition . . . What's harder to accept is that I have passed on this disorder, carried in my genes, to my 11-year-old son."

It hurts Carl to see the difficulties his son already has with even simple tasks. Painful memories linger from his own childhood. Carl remembers how his classmates mimicked and made fun of him, and he worries that Liam's classmates will do the same.

I saw my own life reflected in Carl's emotions. I related to the pure pain a parent feels knowing a life sentence has been passed to a child. I thought of my own parents and a much younger me. There was the day my mother came to spend time with me at Georgetown Hospital in Washington, D.C., shortly after my MS diagnosis. There I lay, flat on my back in a hospital bed, half my face paralyzed with Bell's palsy. I had just lost all vision in one eye from optic neuritis.

My mom felt such anguish that she told me she never would have had children if she had known there was a risk they would inherit MS. Great, Mom, I responded with a chuckle. Thanks a lot. I was not hurt; I only felt bad for her. I told her that my life is not a tragedy. I was happy to be alive and doing well on all the fronts that mattered to me. My determination to stay in motion showed no signs of abating.

My father said little, but over the years it became clear to me how much he struggled with the fact that he had passed along his disease. His mother had done the same to him, of course. I think it was guilt that made the Old Man strangely hard on me. He could be cutting, but I let his occasional critical remarks roll off my back.

One experimental treatment for dystonia is a procedure called deep brain stimulation. DBS involves inserting electrodes into the brain, offering the possibility of substantial improvement in neurological function. The procedure does carry risk. There is some chance of a brain bleed, and there is also the possibility that neurological deficits might worsen.

Because of the risks and his feeling that his symptoms were manageable, Carl had originally intended to wait another five years for DBS. But he changed his mind because Liam's condition was worsening. His son's neurologist recommended that Liam should have the procedure within a year, in hopes that the surgery could help him before his dystonia left him wheelchair-bound. Carl felt compelled to act, feeling he could set an example for Liam. He knew that for his son, the time was right. He knew he had to go under the knife and endure the drill before he could persuade his son to do the same. Carl made clear that he is more focused on Liam's health than his own. "I hope that by taking radical, elective interventions : . . my success will embolden Liam's own courage for the procedure."

"I'm not afraid of this surgery because I have no choice at this point but to sell hope to my son," he wrote to me in an email. "It's hope or bust (death during surgery). I believe hope is the last thing to die, and this hope, expressed as love for family and friends, is all I have left, and now it's tied to DBS."

A follow-up email was necessary because, as I transcribed our phone conversations, I realized I could not understand enough of what Carl was saying. His speech was slurred and disjointed, his voice distorted. I could hear what a strain it was for him to speak.

I knew I had to level with him and thought long and hard about just what to write in my email.

Carl immediately responded. "Thank you for acknowledging my own frustration with my voice," Carl wrote back. "I hope to speak again, and sing again freely. I have a renewed flirtation with the external world."

The DBS procedure takes five to seven hours and is painless. Though the procedure is arduous, it has a space-age appeal. After the anesthetic is administered, a hole is drilled into the skull through which a wire containing four electrodes is inserted. When the electrodes are activated, the impulses emitted are supposed to deactivate the portion of the brain causing the movement malfunctions.

"I recall being awake and in a head frame," Carl said, describing the procedure to me. "I was completely aware of what was going on. I remember the dial my neurologist used to advance the electrodes as he mapped where [they] would benefit the most. I knew there would be a follow-up treatment."

I asked Carl to describe any changes since the initial treatment. We were communicating by email. I was dying to hear Carl's voice, to hear if he had improved. "My body is upright.

It would tend to twist slightly at the neck level and there are less tremors. This overall impact has helped my speech as muscles trigger other muscles (like a dysfunctional network)."

That offered the perfect opening to ask about Carl's garbled words. What about your speech? I asked. "My speech has improved, although my tongue and facial muscles still contract. I have much less fatigue when talking."

And what about Liam? How did he react? "My outcome makes him more optimistic for his own surgery." He left it at that. I felt that Carl was downplaying any real excitement coming from Liam. "As his foot, ankle and calf painfully contract, and I massage it every night, he is in that stage of desperation . . . and social isolation is creeping in. He wasn't able to bike to school with his friends because his 'foot would be too tired to make the ride back.'"

I asked if Liam was going to undergo DBS. "He will. It is tentatively scheduled for six weeks from now." Carl sounded so matter-of-fact. I try to imagine a young boy, strapped down, his head in a cage, knowing that mysterious strangers in gowns and masks are sticking foreign objects into his brain. I think I would be screaming for someone to get me out of there.

"Liam is nervous. He wants to be 'out' for the procedure. I am researching DBS for kids and connecting with parents who have children that underwent the surgery. Yes, we are all scared. It's brain surgery. But Liam can be spared of the progression and that is where we hold our hope."

I had asked Carl if I could talk to Liam about his hopes for the future. When I called, we spoke first about his reaction to being diagnosed with dystonia. Talking to a ten-year-old about such a serious subject is sobering. "Even though I suspected it, it still was a shock," Liam said. "I kind of knew it was there, but I didn't want to believe it. When I was diagnosed, it really hit me hard."

Though his words were stark, Liam's voice sounded even and unemotional. I wondered if the boy really was that calm. Carl had told me Liam has an old soul. Maybe that is a side effect of dystonia, because I heard in his voice the same courage and steadiness that children afflicted with serious diseases often develop.

"Hope is what gets me to move forward," Liam said to me. "Hope that I can be like my dad and get a job and take care of the family—and that I can get it cured. And someday, I don't know, that it won't affect me as much as it is affecting my dad." I enjoyed talking to Liam, and I was very interested to talk to Carl on the phone after his surgery. I wanted to hear his voice and note any changes. I knew how badly he wanted to feel normal and reconnect with the world. I tried for weeks and had trouble reaching him. I began to wonder if Carl was avoiding me. Maybe the improvements had been overstated.

The phone rang late one afternoon. It was Carl. The phone call was stunning. Carl's voice was clear, his enunciation much improved. The sound was not perfect but perfectly understandable. I found the conversation breathtaking. I asked if he thought his life was going to change.

"Yes," Carl responded, "but it's hard to rejoice because Liam is getting worse." I could hear the pain in Carl's voice. "Liam is at a point of desperation. There is a lot of pain at school. At the end of the day, if he could do the DBS tomorrow, he would." Carl paused. "But Liam is scared."

Liam would be given general anesthesia, which generally is not how the procedure is done. I asked Carl if the patient needs to be awake so he can respond to commands from the doctor. "That's right," Carl responded. Then why will Liam be asleep? "That's a good question," Carl answered. We left it at that.

But when we spoke again, the news was very good. Toward the end of 2017, I contacted Carl to ask if Liam had undergone Deep Brain Stimulation. He had, and Carl's email had a new energy. "Liam is biking every day. He used to have to watch the neighborhood kids bike to school without him. Just last week he biked to school for the first time and is using the skateboard he wanted to destroy last year. He's catching up on lost childhood. We hope it halts any progression (but it appears to be doing that). Now he's just a smart-aleck seventh grader, who I'm finally optimistic about." It is heartening to encounter a happy ending.

I remember how small and vulnerable my kids were at Liam's age. Serious sickness is not for the fainthearted. Many families are drawn close by medical crises. Others are torn asunder. Outsiders cannot guess where the winds will blow. I know only that these are good people, strong and resilient. They are hopeful and committed to one another.

Families always should hope for that. Meredith and I have been fortunate. In 2015, Ben, our oldest, returned from nearly four years of living in China. When Ben had settled back in, as part of his preparation for business school he studied coding, a systematic method for analyzing data and generating insights into consumer needs.

Unbeknownst to us, as his coding project, Ben chose the task of identifying and analyzing handicapped-accessible entrances to the New York City subway system. He went about it quietly, telling us nothing about what he was doing. When he showed us the video of his presentation, we were very surprised. And moved. Meredith and I understood his motivation. Clearly Ben, who is now twenty-nine, hoped he could make a difference for me—since I still occasionally use the subway—and for many others.

Gabe, our middle child at twenty-seven, has also made MS his cause. When he worked as a television reporter in Spokane, before moving to his current job in Seattle, he was interviewed at his station about a local MS walk. After explaining that MS is a progressive disease, he told the interviewer, "It moves forward, and we take a step back. This walk is our chance to go forward. Let MS move back."

Lily, now twenty-five years old, ran a half marathon in New York City recently to raise funds for MS. Defiance in the face of debilitating illness is fueled by hope. Our children seem to have a clear path to that hope.

In the end, all of us must grapple with hope. "Hope is being able to see that there is light," Desmond Tutu said, "despite all of the darkness." A family can provide a soft glow for a struggling member. Sometimes, a harsher beam is required.

In moments when I was hurting and hard on those around me, Meredith would set me straight, telling me I was never alone in that hospital bed. She and our three kids were there with me. We endure together, and when a family member is sick, hope moves to high alert. We hope as one. Nothing more needs to be said among us.

CHAPTER 5

Resisting Help

L ily is right about you," Meredith told me several years ago. Lily might be our youngest, but she is definitely not a child any longer. Lily usually is more outspoken, more ready to buck authority than her older brothers are. I had a suspicion where Meredith was going with this.

In recent years, whenever Lily was home and heard me having one of my outbursts over my inability to tie a tie or tuck in a shirt or whatever my latest frustration, she would give me a lecture. I never wanted to hear it because I knew she was right.

"You have to learn to ask for help," Lily had lectured me on a recent visit. "Stop making everyone around you miserable." We had paid for college, but now suddenly she was my mother. I'm not yelling at anyone else, Lily, I protested, only at myself. I just need to let off steam. Lily was not buying it.

I guess I was not either. I knew I was in a grand funk and needed to snap out of it. The eruptions were getting old.

It is difficult to ask for help when all I wish for is a life of my own invention. I wish for a life in which I am free to rise as high as my talents allow. I crave limitless possibilities. MS is a weight I do not want to carry. If I dare to hope, it will be for that burden to be lifted. Times were tough, and I was having trouble locating my red cape.

One evening, I fell. I silently slumped to the floor of my office at our home in a small village on the Hudson River. It was a slow-motion pitch forward that could not be stopped. I crumpled, sinking on legs gone soft, unable to finish the job of crossing the room.

I lay still, looking around for something solid to support my weight—a bedpost or the railing at the top of the stairs. I needed something sturdy to grab and pull myself up. I lifted my deadened right leg into position to help me stand, but I was unable even to get to my knees. I dragged myself along a rug that burned my skin with every pull forward.

My strength was sapped. Finally, I gave up and did what I had wanted to avoid at all costs. I yelled for Meredith. Then I remembered she was downstairs and would not hear me. I crawled to a desk and reached up, knocking a telephone to the floor so I could call her on her cell phone. I knew how upset Meredith was going to be.

Meredith is small and I am tall, not a good recipe for

strenuous teamwork. This time she strained her back trying to lift me to no avail. Her discomfort was obvious. I squirmed with guilt for causing such pain. "What if this happens when I am traveling for work? What will you do then?" The predictable questions came fast and furious.

My mind flashed to happy, peaceful times from our past, like our determined runs through Chicago's Lincoln Park Zoo in subzero temperatures. I remembered hikes up ski slopes in summer, Ben in a backpack, egging me on. Days were long once, nights longer. We owned our lives, and we were happy.

"I'm calling the police," Meredith suddenly announced. "I can't do this anymore. I just can't." A few minutes later, two very large men in uniform presented themselves. Of course, when you're flat-out and smelling the floor, everyone looks particularly large. The cops were affable and effective. Seconds later, they had me on my feet and I was walking normally, at least for me. Just another boring evening at home.

I could not stop wondering why this stuff happens to some of us. Why me? I always resist asking that question. It has the sound of a victim. Maybe the only answer is "Why not me?"

I understand illness and injury arrive indiscriminately. Still, I could not let go of the "Why me?" question, though I kept my obsession to myself. Following a series of emails, I was able to arrange a meeting with Rabbi Harold Kushner, who had written a seminal book addressing that age-old question.

When Bad Things Happen to Good People spoke to the many living with loss.

Rabbi Kushner generously agreed to meet with me and suggested a day when we could convene at his temple office in the suburban town of Natick, about twenty miles from Boston, where he is now rabbi laureate.

My taxi delivered me to Temple Israel, where I was shown to a seat outside the rabbi's study. Soon a white-haired gentleman arrived and ushered me into his study. The rabbi looked great for his eighty-one years. He was tall and dignified. His old study, on the other hand, was not so elegant. The space had the look of a small abandoned warehouse.

The simple surroundings made sense. Rabbi Kushner was an unpretentious man. He made me feel comfortable at once. He was warm and not at all reluctant to talk about the sensitive subject he knew I was there to discuss. Instead of speaking about my MS, I wanted to hear about the rabbi's own loss. In November 1966, on the very day that their daughter was born, Harold and his wife Suzette's three-year-old son, Aaron, was diagnosed with progeria, or "rapid aging," a rare genetic disorder. The disease strikes one in eight million babies. Aaron died when he was fourteen.

How do you make sense of what you went through with the death of your son? I asked. His answer was simple. "You don't. You don't even try," he responded evenly. "It is truly random."

Rabbi Kushner told me he expected only friends and family to read *When Bad Things Happen to Good People*. Instead, it was a runaway bestseller, remaining on the *New York Times* list for eighteen months. The book became a bible for the many who knew personal pain.

"I wanted to write a book that could be given to the person who has been hurt by life," the rabbi wrote in his introduction, "by death, by illness or injury, by rejection or disappointment—and who knows in his heart that if there is justice in the world, he deserved better."

Rabbi Kushner made it clear that he believes the pain we suffer in life often is arbitrary. "Some people have good luck for no reason. Some have bad luck." He then acknowledged my health problems. "You understand that and I understand that." He added that he does not blame God. "It's not God's job to make sick people healthy. It's God's job to make sick people brave."

The rabbi sat back in an old desk chair and began speaking softly. "You don't have any control over whether this is going to happen to you or not," he told me. "You've got a lot of control over what you are going to do about it. You can respond with grace and courage, or you can respond with despair and the search for somebody to blame. That is up to you."

In *When Bad Things Happen to Good People*, Rabbi Kushner says that such an opportunity to respond to adversity is a gift. For him, writing the book was a chance to make a highly personal statement, to "distill some blessing out of Aaron's pain and tears."

I felt a new energy as he spoke. Even when he was talking about his own experience, it was like he was talking about my life. "Let me suggest that the bad things that happen to us in our lives do not have a meaning when they happen to us," Rabbi Kushner went on. "They do not happen for any good reason that would cause us to accept them willingly. But we can give them meaning. We can redeem these tragedies from senselessness by imposing meaning on them."

In other words, *it is up to us to make sense out of what happens and give it meaning.* To do that is an achievement. His sentiment was echoed by a passage I had read and tucked away by Václav Havel, the Czech writer and first president of the Czech Republic. "Hope is . . . not the conviction that something will turn out well, but the certainty that something makes sense, regardless of how it turns out."

How many of us possess the emotional strength to will that certainty into being? I asked the rabbi. "There are people who have had the hope just bled out of them, and I pity them," Rabbi Kushner said. But he seemed to think such people are the exceptions. "The average person, give them any tiny crack of light, and they will fasten on to that. It is self-fulfilling to a very great degree."

Rabbi Kushner offered a final thought. "The real takeaway

is that no matter how unfair life is, God gives us the resources to handle it. And God gives us people to make sure we never feel abandoned and alone."

On the train back to New York, I replayed our conversation on my digital recorder. I felt that the rabbi had offered me punctuation for my inquiry, a period to place after the last sentence. I was grateful; I had grown tired of question marks.

I am grateful for the family that has put up with so much from me and for the friends I can talk to, those who understand the questions I ask. Whether or not it is God's gift, to not feel abandoned and alone may be the best we can hope for in this life.

One day, I fell one time too many. Meredith wanted to call the police again. Her words fell on deaf ears. I shouted, no, please don't. I was upset and insisting I would get myself up. I all but banished her from the room. Not a smart move. I was out of control and more self-conscious about bothering the police again than about what I was doing to my wife.

Meredith had a different take on the situation. She had been pushed over the edge. She angrily told me she was done with the MS. I still can visualize the desperation on her face. "We can't live this way," she kept repeating. I was not to ask her to do anything more for me. Period.

Meredith added that some of our friends thought I was

selfish, thinking only of myself. Then she abruptly left the house. Meredith was pissed and probably hurt. This was a sobering moment for me. I thought hard about how much Meredith does for me and how ungrateful I must seem, nursing my own emotional needs and ignoring hers.

It took me more than an hour to pull myself up three stairs toward her office so that I could use the iron railing to help me stand. Finally, I was vertical. I knew I had to do something about my attitude. My self-absorption had reached critical mass. I sat at the computer and consulted Dr. Google to find a company that sells pendants with a button to send an alarm when there is a medical emergency.

After ordering the pendant, I took a deep breath and contacted the local constabulary. It was time to have a conversation with them. As usual, the men in blue were terrific. I don't know why I was so hesitant to involve them. They told me they go to people's homes regularly to assist residents in need. "There is an elderly lady with MS who falls out of her wheelchair almost every day," one officer explained in a reassuring tone. "We are always there."

The officers agreed to take a key to the front door in case Meredith was away when I paid one of my visits to the floor. They put me at ease, but they kept calling me "sir." I thought of what they had said about the old lady who could not stay in her wheelchair, and I figured the young cops must have seen me as an old man.

I knew I could not let vanity get in my way. I had waited far too long to make these moves. When you are acutely ill, self-absorption may be excusable. Maybe. But I had strayed from understanding that when it results from a chronic disease, sorry, Charlie. Chronic illness is a family affair. Spouses have the burden of tending to the needs of a loved one, even when they would secretly rather push him out a window. I knew they should not be treated as spectators when they are in the ring with us.

It's funny how self-absorption can marry self-doubt. They feed off each other. More than forty years since the diagnosis, I was feeling more threatened than ever. I was scared silly of finding myself in a helpless state from which there would be no escape. It scared me that my deterioration was outpacing my father's.

No longer could I slide smoothly into the front passenger seat of a car; instead, I had to grab my leg with my hands and drag the deadened limb into the vehicle. One day I realized I could not move my fingers enough to put on a pair of gloves. I stared at my right hand in disbelief. I could not write or even hold a pen in my right hand. I could not hold a fork with that hand and eat, couldn't shave or brush my teeth with it either. I had to pivot to the left. I was a right-handed guy living a left-handed life.

No longer could I pretend I was winning the war. In short, I was in a bad place, withdrawn and spending too much time alone. One day my home phone rang and rang. Caller ID signaled it was a good friend. I listened to the message. He was inviting me to join him to walk along the river, as we so often did.

My chest tightened, but I did not answer. I waited until the message finished and then erased it. I only wanted to be left alone. I was hiding, warehousing myself on a dusty shelf out of sight.

This was the condition I found myself in during the spring of 2012, when Meredith called from the car on her way home from work to tell me she had been contacted about a stem cell conference to be held at the Vatican. The two of us were going to be invited to participate.

Huh? This was intriguing, since Rome is among our favorite places and, at the very least, it would be wonderful to have a reason to go there again. But the proposed plan was also puzzling. The Vatican hosting a seminar analyzing stem cell therapies? Meredith went on to say that they wanted her to act as one of the overall hosts, and they were interested in having me chair a panel on cell therapy and its applications for autoimmune diseases, including MS. Of course, that was a subject about which I knew precisely nothing. Weird. What was this all about? I wondered. I could hear Meredith shrug over the phone.

When we hung up, I sat in silence for a few minutes. I struggled to make sense of a stem cell conference at the Vatican. The Catholic Church's fierce opposition to embryonic stem cell research was well known. The idea of my participation at such a gathering was also confusing, since I could not imagine what I would bring to it.

But the prospect of a scientific meeting shedding light on stem cell therapy certainly was enticing. I had not known that patients were already being treated with stem cells. Could this be a ticket out of my cave? A trip to Rome sounded pretty good too. I was excited, even a little bit hopeful about what I might learn there. A seed had been planted in my head. I needed to hear more.

CHAPTER 6

The Invitation

L ate one chilly December afternoon in 2012, Meredith, her assistant Brooke, and I crossed town to the Graybar Building, the old office complex adjoining Grand Central Station. We had been asked to meet with Dr. Robin Smith, a physician who was working closely with high-level Vatican officials to plan the conference on adult stem cell therapy.

I wanted to learn how this emerging medical technology was being used to improve the lives of those living with chronic illnesses, including MS. We were in teeming midtown Manhattan, and everywhere we looked there were people carrying Christmas packages. We eagerly cut through the crowds and headed for the meeting.

Soon after our arrival, we were ushered into a large conference room where Dr. Smith and several of her associates joined us. From the moment she walked into the room, it was clear that Dr. Smith—Robin—was a force to be reckoned with. She had the meeting up and running immediately after introductions were made. A urologist by training, Robin is CEO of NeoStem, a publicly traded stem cell company and president of the Stem for Life Foundation, the cosponsor—along with the Vatican—of the Rome conference.

As Robin described the conference agenda and schedule, her confidence and comfort level with the Vatican, that mysterious city within a city, were evident. The conference would take place in April 2013, she said. Robin had anticipated what our concerns might be and had planned every detail of our proposed six-night stay in Rome.

She shared strong opinions about whom we should meet and get to know. She told us what roles we were expected to fulfill and even what parts our children might play if they wanted to join the expedition to Italy.

As the room buzzed with talk of logistics and arrangements, Robin came over to sit next to me. Lowering her voice so that only I could hear, she leaned into me. "You are going to meet many individuals involved with all kinds of cell therapies," she said. "And I know others who are not going to Rome whom I can introduce you to as well." I looked hard at her. What was she telling me? "I want you to know I am committed to getting you treated. I think I can make that happen."

I was taken aback. I had known this woman for about an hour and had no reason to expect a gesture like that. Robin's take-charge manner had softened as she spoke to me, and her sincerity was clear. I was touched. My appreciation of her kindness was eclipsed only by my quiet excitement at the prospect of finding help.

Suddenly something very new was happening in my head. A forty-year period of knowing no hope of regaining health was beginning to give way to feelings I could not even identify. An actual physical sensation I never had felt, a kind of tingling up and down my spine, caused me to squirm slightly in my seat.

As I silently struggled to mull over exactly what Robin had just offered, she switched back to her efficiency mode and began speaking to the room again. Embryonic stem cells were no longer the cells of choice for most medical research, she explained. Adult cells now were more commonly used. I had not known that, but it did begin to explain why the Vatican was comfortable hosting a stem cell conference.

She went on to explain how most of the trillions of cells in our bodies have well-formed architecture and only function in specific parts of the body. But stem cells are super cells, blank slates. These undesignated cells have the potential to morph into many different cell types, ready to become whatever is needed to assist healing in a body damaged by disease. While embryonic stem cells can assume an unlimited range of tissue types, adult stem cells have a more limited range. They can morph into any type of cell of the organ from which they came.

Given scientists' ability to manipulate them in uniform ways, stem cells have been useful in testing new drugs, but their more direct and exciting application is cell-based therapies.

In theory, these cells can provide solutions for conditions in which healthy cells have been killed or damaged. They might be used to create new organs and decrease our dependence on donated organs.

Their regenerative powers also could be effective in treating conditions such as macular degeneration, diabetes, and spinal cord injuries. And, as Robin Smith suggested, multiple sclerosis.

In patients with multiple sclerosis, the body's immune system has turned on itself and attacked the myelin sheath insulating the central nervous system. Without this insulation, the cells of the brain, spinal cord, and optic nerves can short-circuit. Researchers hope that stem cells will be able to morph into cell types to repair or replace those that MS has damaged or destroyed.

In theory, stem cells can repair old wounds. Individuals who have languished in wheelchairs for years have been known to stand and walk again. There is no formula for second-guessing what cell therapy might accomplish. Damage to the body from accidents may be different from the loss of function from a disease process. We are in the earliest years of stem cell therapy. That makes all of us laboratory rats.

Back on that day in 2012, I found myself having trouble concentrating as Robin continued. My mind kept wandering back to our private conversation. Had I heard Robin accurately when she sounded so sure of herself, almost promising my MS would be treated? I could not imagine where, when, or how that would happen, but her confidence was contagious. I was experiencing technical difficulties, trying to slow down my runaway mind. I was not the obsessive type but certainly was making an exception at this moment.

As my attention came back to the room again, I heard her explaining that the Catholic Church wanted to use the conference to move beyond the embryonic stem cell controversy and showcase its support for research with adult cells. A previous stem cell conference had been planned for 2010 but was canceled when invited scientists accused the Church of trying to censor them. She promised the new conference would let the world know that change was coming to the Holy See.

Meredith and I looked at each other. Red flags went up in our minds. I said nothing, but my distrust of organized religion was deep and had been since I'd abandoned faith in my youth. Even if the controversy over the embryonic cells issue was pushed aside, I could not help wondering if it really had been resolved.

Regardless of our reservations about the Vatican's stance, Robin was determined that this conference succeed, and she had given much thought to choosing the participants to make such success a reality. The cast included scientists and opinion leaders, philanthropists and journalists. Robin wanted Meredith, well known for her work in the news business and as an advocate for MS causes, to act as conference host at the first session.

She also wanted me to chair the opening panel, which would address stem cell therapy and autoimmune disorders, including multiple sclerosis. This proposed role scared me to death. I had nothing erudite to say about this weighty subject. I was not sure I even could pronounce *myelin*.

I was reassured to learn the plan was for me to open the gathering not by explaining the science of stem cell therapy but by describing the patient experience of illness. That I could do. I would then act as traffic cop for the participants on the panel I was moderating as they engaged with the audience.

Robin said there would be two scientists on my panel: Richard Burt, chief of Immunotherapy and Autoimmune Diseases in the Department of Medicine at Northwestern University in Chicago, and Saud Sadiq, director and chief research scientist at the Tisch MS Research Center in New York. With participants of that caliber, the conference would be compelling. There would be new ideas in the air, presented by world-class physicians and scientists.

They wouldn't have to try too hard to sell me on the science. I realized I would do anything a scientist suggested, take any chance. I was ready to take any experimental drug and felt no fear. I had been waiting for an opportunity like this for more decades than I cared to count. This would be my moment.

My thoughts and the tingling in my spine continued, startling in their intensity and immediacy. They almost were reminiscent of drug trips during my college years. Mouths were moving in the conference room, but I was hearing words as white noise. I was having sensory overload, and my thoughts had turned inward.

One dimension of my life—which I never discussed and rarely acknowledged even to myself—is the terror that grips me when I consider growing old with an illness that is going to keep exacting a greater and greater toll on me. When I close my eyes, I see the outlines of a white cane and wheelchair in my future. To me, those are symbols of surrender, the tools of defeat for a failing body that has been decimated by disease and can fight no more. I fear helplessness above all. I have always understood that this disease process cannot be stopped. But could stem cell therapy work for me? Might I actually be treated and cured by one of these doctors? Sooner or later someone will be cured of MS. Why not me?

I found myself viewing my future life through a gauze filter. The white cane and wheelchair had disappeared from the snapshot developing in my mind. I was picturing my body being restored, being whole again. I had made the quantum leap to a cure through revolutionary treatments that were still untested and unproven.

The caution I had learned as a journalist fell away as my imagination raced ahead. I was not tempted to turn back. No way. I knew precious little about the emerging field of cell therapy—I had heard about it only moments before. I did not care. That strange feeling was still pulsating through my body. Could this be what hope felt like?

My attention was jerked back to the conference room again, this time when Robin asked if I knew Dr. Sadiq. In fact, I did. I explained I had met with him briefly in the past on a matter that had nothing to do with my illness. I had liked him. Liking a neurologist was a headline with me, I told her. I had been impressed by Dr. Sadiq because he seemed to have an open mind, which struck me as unusual.

I had never met Dr. Burt, but I learned that he was already treating patients with some sort of cell therapy. I wondered if he would take me on as a patient. Perhaps I could receive treatment as a perquisite for my work at the conference. In hindsight, this was all insane. My imagination was working overtime; my brain, hardly at all.

Leaving Robin's office that night, our steps echoed through the deserted lobby. The emptiness of the post–rush hour building seemed to cast a pall on us. We had been grappling with a serious subject. No one took it lightly. But I, of course, had taken the subject and blasted off into outer space.

Meredith and her assistant kept glancing at me, as if they were hearing what was going on in my head. If they had noticed me zoning out as Robin talked and were waiting for me to tell them how I was feeling, I did not cooperate. I kept my thoughts to myself and a neutral expression on my face. I did not mean to be coy. It just was too soon to talk.

My head was throbbing, replaying the videotape of the afternoon's gathering at full volume. I was hearing trumpets blaring, a chorus singing, and I felt hypnotized by the music. I could not shake that strange physical sensation, and I didn't want to. It was like finding God when I did not even know he was lost.

CHAPTER 7

Leaving Conventional Care

E arly in the new millennium, I had battled colon cancer twice. The disease knocked me down hard. This
was out of bounds, I thought. I already had my disease. I was indemnified against getting hit by another. Right?
Wrong. The word *cancer* touched off a maelstrom that sucked
the entire family under. When cancer comes calling, you find
out what you are made of. By the time I had my second bout
with cancer, I got my answer, and it was not pretty.

My kids did a lot of growing up in the next year. They
learned that life is not fair. The three of them saw me morph
into an angry man they did not know, and they figured out
how to deal with it. Each of them learned about stress and
emotional pain on a whole new level. Meredith and I followed
our self-imposed guidelines and sat the kids down, quietly
using the *C*-word. Gabe spoke up first, asking if I was going
to die, quickly followed by a request for clarification about the

disposition of holiday presents. Clearly, Gabe's priorities were in order.

In the first case, the surgeon went in through my lower back, removing the coccyx, or tailbone. The post-op pain was searing. The second time, the cancer was still harder to reach. The surgeon warned me he might have to do a temporary ileostomy, which would mean I would need the bag. The bag. Great. The prospect of that worried me more than the cancer itself. I knew trouble lay in wait.

The surgery lasted almost seven hours. I awoke with a port on my arm to deliver morphine and a bag on my belly. Don't worry, I was told, the bag was temporary. The procedure would probably be reversed in three or four months. Long ago, MS had taught me to count on nothing. I knew not to trust the word *probably*. All I could do was desperately hope the arrangement really was temporary and just grit my teeth and live with the indignity.

When I returned home from the hospital, the autumn chill moved indoors, my anger arriving under the cover of my darkness. This was not supposed to happen. Did I mention that life is unfair? I could not get used to that simple fact. I was pissed and acting half my age. The kids bore the brunt of my anger. I thought they would rejoice that I was home again. Instead they shrank in horror. I moved around the house with a trail of black smoke behind me.

My fangs were bared, and they were sharp. Do your

homework! Turn off the music! I barked. Clean up that mess! Don't leave it for your mother and me.

Cohabitating with my MS had seemed simple by comparison. Now the children were walking on eggshells, never sure of what might touch off the next explosion. I was trapped in my own despair.

Finally, Meredith made it plain she had seen enough. "You are becoming a monster," she bluntly told me. "These are your children." I just sat and stared, seeming oblivious but taking her seriously. My bad mood had built up a lot of inertia, however, and change came slowly.

When the ileostomy finally was reversed, the bottom of my colon kept closing, and the painful complications got worse. I was impossible to be around. "Open your eyes, Richard," my wife pleaded. "Don't do this to your children. You are not in this alone."

Memories from this period carry pure pain. It was as if my children were the real victims of my cancer. I thought my love for them had no borders, but I was hurting them every day. Meredith's pleas to me finally hit home. I had to do something, anything to change course.

I sat each of the kids down individually and told them I wanted to write about this awful situation. I wanted them to see my mea culpa in black and white, no holds barred. I told the kids they would have to be honest with me, and they could say anything. My editor at *The New York Times* had agreed to the piece and told me it would run as a Cases column in the Science section.

Ben, you are thirteen, I said quietly. You can tell me the truth. Have I been hard to live with? Ben smiled suspiciously and sat, just staring at me. "Do you really want the truth?" he asked. My blood ran cold as I wondered what he was going to throw at me.

The floodgates opened. "You were really mean," he began, pleased to unload and picking up steam. "I wanted to scream in your face and kick you. But Mom told me to cut you some slack."

These were sobering statements. Gabe, who was then eleven, added his two painful cents when it was his turn. "It sounded like you really hate us," he said. A flood of emotions was cascading in. I knew I had to go through this exercise, but it hurt.

Lily was still little, not quite ten. She simply wagged her finger in silent disapproval. Their pain had been dumped at my feet. What had I done? Even formulating words to apologize caused me anguish. An improved domestic landscape would require more than words anyway. The epiphany hit hard. I had been so self-absorbed, and there was a lot more to think about than me.

I had lost the ability to see my family through my veil of self-absorption and pain. I did not realize what I was doing because I was the center of my universe. What I missed was a simple fact. Patients do not lie alone in their hospital beds. Our families are next to us, whether or not we see them.

On the day of my endless surgery, Ben had played in a violin recital at school. His music teacher later told me she had rarely heard so much raw emotion come out of a child's violin.

It is easy for us parents to reassure ourselves that the kids are used to bumps in the road and have their acts together. Dream on.

Once I had beaten back the beast, MS took its turn again. Multiple sclerosis moves in when the body is most vulnerable. Various appendages began to fail with un-nerving frequency. I subjected myself to one drug regimen after another in the hope of reversing or at least stemming the steady slippage of my physical abilities.

In previous years, one of my neurologists recommended taking three injections of interferon every week. I then gradu-ated to daily injections of a different drug. By my count, I plunged needles into various fleshy spots on my body nearly one thousand times. I never complained, but I also never got used to the exercise. The interferon and other drugs did noth-ing to stop the progress of the illness. They were not even in-tended to do battle with my brand of multiple sclerosis, secondary progressive MS, but the neurologist thought they were worth trying.

There are no treatments for SPMS. Neurologists often treat people who have this form of the disease with drugs intended for the more common relapsing remitting disease to see if the pharmaceuticals help. That is called a Hail Mary pass. In my case, the drugs for RRMS never worked.

I have to wonder if physicians can hit the broad side of a barn at point-blank range when firing at MS. And really, what are they shooting at, anyway? Even in the body of one patient, they may be aiming at limbs or lesions on the brain or perhaps an optic nerve or two. My own body has seen the best and brightest take aim and fire. We need to believe in and trust our physicians. Hope cannot thrive without trust. These men and women are devoted to finding cause and cure. I know that. They are good people. It is not fair to label them the gang that can't shoot straight, but that doesn't make it any easier to accept that nothing was working.

After my battle with cancer I was impatient, ready to try any treatment, no matter the side effects. I decided to change neurologists. Mine were friends but too conservative for me. I wanted action.

I had a long relationship with the big MS guy at Harvard. In 2009, I asked him to take me on as a patient and think outside the box. Chemotherapy was his recommendation. Oy. Doctors cannot be faulted for following a patient's wishes and throwing everything they can at a disease. Sometimes that helps. Many times it does not. Nothing ventured, nothing gained, though there is certainly a point when the treatment feels as bad as the illness.

My experiment with chemo was devastating. Each month, I walked into the cancer infusion center at a major New York medical center. Every treatment day brought the same drill. An IV of Benadryl came first, intended to ward off the harsh reactions to the chemo that would show up anyway. The antihistamine did make me pleasantly sleepy, but then the real poisoning began. After about an hour on the Cytoxan, a powerful form of chemo used to battle various cancers by slowing or stopping cell growth, my body started shaking violently. A few blankets later, I still was freezing. This went on month after month.

Every time, I just wanted to get up and sprint out of there, as if that would have been possible. Cancer patients, hairless and gaunt, sick and dying, surrounded me. I could not stop looking at them. They were cheerful and warm, smiling at me as if I were one of them. Most seemed upbeat. I wondered if they were optimistic.

While I was undergoing chemo, so was my friend and former colleague Sandor Polster. Sandy had written news copy for both Walter Cronkite and Tom Brokaw for years, but by that point he was writing the last chapter of his life. Sandy was dying of gastric cancer and knew he was running out of time. Polster's chemo sessions had been rugged. Mine were nothing in comparison.

We had lunch in late 2012, and he seemed upbeat, though hardly optimistic. I asked if he had hope. "Yes," he quickly answered. "I hope I outlive my cell phone contract." That was vintage Polster. I kept probing.

What keeps you going? I asked. "I want to get to talk to my grandson. That is my incentive to live. He is one. I do not expect to be alive to have a conversation in two years." Staying alive for that boy sounds like hope, I suggested. "I am going to live life. I guess that's hope, maybe with a lowercase *h*." He added that he wanted his last meal to be an all-you-can-eat buffet. Sandy exited laughing.

After each round of chemo, I rushed home to drink liters of water, hoping to avoid a severe bladder infection. Violent mood swings followed. I would laugh maniacally, only to find myself weeping a few hours later. The reactions were hell. This got old fast. One day when the weather was warm, Meredith and I sat outside, and I found myself explaining through my tears that, really, nothing was wrong.

Actually, chemo was wrong. Big-time. Meredith begged me to get off the poison, which eventually I did. My neurologist was disappointed I gave up on the chemo. A patient cannot be weak-kneed if there is any hope of beating a disease like mine. I felt bad about pulling the plug. But not too bad. The Cytoxan had turned my hair white, but it did not turn around my illness.

My war was with my body, but many battles are fought

north of the neck. Had I hoped the drug would make a difference? I suppose. But my expectation level had moved south to near zero. *Hope* was not an active verb in my life. Hope and expectation have to at least be proportional. They do not need to match perfectly, but they must at least exist in the same space.

In early 2013, I decided I had reached my limit with conventional treatment. There would be no medical miracle. I had endured almost forty years of fruitless treatments, a few so harsh they seemed as debilitating as the MS. I liked my doctors, but I wanted out. I was weary of listening to the predictable expressions of encouragement and hope from the doctors. "Maybe" and "Let's try" are up there with "Someday" and "In the future." "We can hope" is also a favorite. Please.

I was running in place and tired of pretending we were getting somewhere. That was why I told my New York neurologist I was done. I was taking my football and heading home. The doctor understood my frustration. There were no hard feelings. She knew my decision to abandon conventional care was not personal. I just needed space. As I left her office, I told her that when she found a cure to please let me know. She smiled.

I had resigned my commission in the MS militia. I had not been without a neurologist in the four decades since my diagnosis. I felt slightly vulnerable, unprotected, even though

I knew no doctor could shield me from the inevitable decline I was facing. But I was free. No more fruitless forays into territory captured by the neurological enemy. Relief rose inside me. I now was walking the wire with no net, but I felt unburdened, at least for the moment.

I had been bluntly warned by my first neurologist in 1973 that there would be little he could do. All these years later, that tough truth hit me hard. He had dismissed hope in the first five minutes of my new relationship with MS. That raises a tricky question. Are such blunt assessments a sensible plan for helping anyone deal with a life-altering disease? There is nothing positive to be said for dispensing rose-colored fiction. But maybe leaving room for hope could pay off down the line. Who can second-guess tomorrow? Medicine has been on the march for years, developing new drugs and devices. No one, doctor or patient, should discount the future.

Over the years, family and friends talked to me about hope. Hope seemed to be more of a comfort station for them than for me. Hope was not my thing. I saw hope as a hiding place for losers. Winners, I felt, just kept moving forward on their own steam. Little about my attitude with regard to hope had changed. I still was determined to erase hope from my emotional vocabulary.

Meredith thought my move away from regular care a bit impetuous, but basically she got it. I thought going it alone felt fine. But once I let go of any lingering notion that something might fall out of the sky and one day make me better, I didn't feel fine at all. I began to focus entirely on my miseries. I knew I was stuck in a self-indulgent rut. I recognized my emotional cycles, but that did not help me escape them. I was pretty moody.

"You are an angry person, Richard," Meredith told me one day as I sat sulking in the wake of one of my angry explosions. We had been hanging out in our family room, waiting for the evening news to start, when I dropped a coaster on the floor. I had an instant meltdown as my fumbling fingers failed to pick it up. My fits of anger were coming too frequently, and Meredith was growing tired of the show. Meredith is liable to say anything on television, and she certainly speaks her mind at home.

Strong voices at home demand to be heard. The message was received but not yet processed. Criticisms can be pleas for change and gain momentum with repeated soundings. The cumulative effect is only seen over time. Change can take place quietly and without fanfare. A state of being can be silently altered, even without acknowledgment from the party in question.

CHAPTER 8

A Bleak Landscape

By early 2013, I was fed up with conventional treatment and life as patient. Still, the stem cell conference was coming up, and Dr. Burt's new approach remained intriguing—maybe too much so. I began preparing for the conference and at the same time planning strategy for my imminent pitch to Dr. Burt. I read articles about him and watched videos of his work, which he had posted online. I figured I would have one shot with him, and I did not want to blow it. I was going to be ready.

Being treated by Dr. Burt was already a done deal as far as I was concerned. I was violating every rule of journalism: jumping to conclusions, predicting outcomes, and exploiting access. Dr. Robin Smith had encouraged me to contact members of my panel to talk about Rome. I had a valid reason to speak to Burt, even if my primary motivation for making the call had nothing to do with the Vatican conference.

When I felt I had perfected the pitch, I called the number Robin had given me, heart in my throat. The doctor was out of the country and would not be reachable for ten days, his receptionist explained. All the adrenaline that had been revving me up suddenly dissipated. I was deflated but determined to hold my act together. This was no time for impatience, and keeping expectations in check became my new priority. I wanted to control the tidal wave of raw emotion that had been turned loose with the prospect of a dramatic reversal.

As I slept that night, I replayed a powerful recurring dream. I fell to the floor of my home and grimly positioned myself to stand. In this iteration of the dream, I shocked myself by standing with no apparent effort. I then walked briskly to find Meredith and deliver the good news.

Was this home movie a glimpse into the future or just another silly scenario of wishful thinking? Was it really possible that I might return to jogging in the park? I knew I should not allow myself to, but as I counted down the days until my conversation with Dr. Burt, I took a brief holiday from caution. This fantasy was all I had.

The day Dr. Burt's receptionist had suggested I contact him arrived. I called. Burt was not there but soon contacted me. "Mr. Cohen, this is Dr. Burt. How can I help you?" said the voice on the other end of the line. A chill wind blew through the receiver.

Dr. Burt seemed a bit disengaged, even impatient. Maybe

he was tired. We talked about Rome only briefly. I could tell this was going to be a short conversation and realized that if I was going to bring up the subject of a possible stem cell transplant or something, I had better do it fast. Out it came in a rush of words. After he asked me a few questions about my history and age, he delivered a quick response. "I assume you have secondary progressive disease and probably have had multiple sclerosis for too long. I cannot help you." And then he hung up. The iceman goeth.

I tried to hide my disappointment, but it was obvious to Meredith. "I'm sorry" was all she said. She could have added *dumb shit*, but she didn't. She realized how much I had riding on that call. It was clear, even to me, that I had gotten way ahead of myself. I felt silly for allowing my expectations to get so out of hand.

True to form, I immediately distanced myself from my emotions and returned to working on a few writing projects. It was as if the dance with the doctor had never happened. My years of dueling with disease had taught me the need for resilience. I knew how to bounce back, but I was weary and almost out of bounce.

When I could take time away from other projects, I continued preparing for the Rome event. One day I went to Robin's office for a conference call with Dr. Sadiq. When we discussed his approach to the upcoming panel at the Vatican, he was as warm as I remembered from our brief meetings years before. Dr. Sadiq was responsive when I asked him about his stem cell research, offering intriguing details about what he was doing. I was careful to make sure that this time my questions really were for the sole purpose of preparing for the conference. In the weeks that followed, Robin regularly sent me articles and journal pieces about the latest research in stem cell therapies. Most were interesting, some incomprehensible. What was clear from all of them was that this was a field of science and medicine coming into its own. Even beyond my initial self-interest, I found this world of change and plans for the conference compelling.

As I was studying, Meredith was preparing to host an NBC News special on regenerative medicine, the process of growing organs from stem cells. I was blown away by her report on how much stem cell therapy was already in practice. I had thought we would be looking into the distant future. There was no need for a crystal ball. Therapies were coming on stream now.

As I continued to read the articles Robin sent, I realized I was not alone in my hope for a better life. Scientists and patients alike were anxious to turn corners they never knew were there. Improved lives waited on the road ahead. Fortunes were changing. Hope was out there somewhere. Every time I thought about the stem cell therapies, that strange tingling sensation washed over me. I liked it. It felt right. But even as I continued to wonder if and when I would be treated, I remained grounded, not allowing myself to bury my head too deep in fantasy again.

Still, after decades of pushing away thoughts of recovered vision and restored mobility, I was allowing promising images in my head some room to play. Whenever I thought about the trip to the Vatican scheduled for April, I felt at least a small surge of hope. I was keenly aware of the irony of a secular Jew seeking salvation at the Vatican. I am not a believer, not even an agnostic. I am an atheist—an equal-opportunity cynic. For most of my life, I have believed that in biblical times, with low life expectancies, people searched for a way to handle their mortality. Scholars became fiction writers and moved to Hollywood, and an industry was born.

My distance from any organized religion, including my own, probably had its roots in my mother's attitudes. My mother was born Roman Catholic. Her religion didn't last beyond her early twenties, when she was a young obstetric nurse at Bellevue, New York's storied city hospital. Working in the hospital's delivery rooms in the mid-1940s, she would see the same poor Irish women, overweight and often toothless, come in year after year to deliver the latest additions to their growing families. They were such regulars that their names were well known on the floors.

Each time these mothers and their infants were discharged, the nurses would call out to them as they headed home, "See you next year, dearie." My mother regarded their constant pregnancies as the fault of the Church's opposition to birth control. At ninety-four, my mother still sounded angry when the subject of the Church and women was raised. "I really had no use for the Catholic Church," she told me. Except for occasional weddings and funerals, my mother never set foot in a Catholic church again. When my mom died in 2016, she remained unrepentant.

Her dismissal of the Catholic Church was openly discussed in the family, and distrust of organized religion seemed to be in my DNA. Even as a young person, I believed that, in biblical times, with low life expectancies, the masses searched for a way to explain away their mortality. Old Testament thinkers became fiction writers and moved to Hollywood, giving birth to a new industry.

My father was Jewish. When he met my mother, he was chief resident in anesthesiology at Bellevue. My mother worked in one of the operating rooms where he practiced. They saw no future together—her flaming red hair was like a "Kiss me, I'm Irish" sign—but did not stop flirting. In the 1940s, before air-conditioning, according to one oft-quoted story, my father complained about the heat in the OR and asked my mother to open a window. "While you are up," he said in a loud voice, "feel free to jump out."

My mother told the other nurses there was no way the two of them could have a life together. Intermarriage was heresy in those days. Still, it became a little less rare when, against the odds, a City of New York justice of the peace married my parents on July 2, 1945.

My father's Russian Jewish relatives had no problem with the union. His parents were busy with their own dysfunctional relationship. My mother's Irish Catholic family was appalled and all but disowned her. Only when children arrived did peace slowly return to the family. Religion was not an easy subject at family reunions.

My parents made a half-hearted attempt at Reform Judaism for me and my siblings. My father dragged his feet when it came to arranging religious training for us. Finally, my mother told him to join a temple or we would be in church very soon. That was never going to happen, but we were dispatched to Sunday school soon enough.

My indifference to religion was complete at a tender age. When it was time, my father raised the issue of bar mitzvahs, first to my older brother, then to me. My brother was told the ceremony would be a family affair and would not be turned into the social event of the season. My brother, no fool, said no thanks. I was in my me-too phase and did not have to be asked twice.

As a family, the only time we embraced religion was at holidays. We got together with my father's side of the family during the High Holidays and at Hanukkah and Passover, and we gathered around the Christmas tree with our Irish kin. I thought this was the best of both worlds. If we were festive Jews, I was a restive Jew. I was comfortable with my cultural identity and never questioned my lack of faith.

Meredith was brought up as a Catholic, though her mother had a prickly relationship with the local church. Meredith had wandered away from her religion by the time I met her. She does not go to church often but does not like to be called a lapsed Catholic. In later years she was deeply offended by the pedophile priest scandals. Meredith says she believes in God but has made her disdain for organized religion well known. So you tell me. Obviously, ours is a marriage made somewhere south of heaven.

Regardless of being a nonbeliever, I had no emotional stake in criticizing the Church, however, and at the moment, the reverse was true. I intended to lay off my cynicism. I figured it was time to cut the Church some slack, since the evolving science that interested me suggested I play by Rome's rules. Fair enough.

When we arrived in Rome, I would set aside harsh judgments.

While there would be no articles of faith packed in my suitcase, no appeals to God as I passed through the gates of the Holy See, I would try to be open to whatever miracles might be wrought—though I assumed they would arrive courtesy of science, not God. If nothing came of the conference—as nothing had come of so many drugs, devices, and dreams—at least we would eat well in Italy.

CHAPTER 9

Hope as a Family Affair

Despite my discomfort with establishment religion, I am comfortable with my cultural identity. It's cool to be a Jew, as long as you hold it down to Hanukkah and Passover, with an occasional nod to Rosh Hashanah, the Jewish New Year. Actually I have a deep respect for Jewish literature, history, and music. I knew I wanted to talk to religious leaders about hope. Jews will think anything to death. It was the inevitable death of a child, the daughter of a female rabbi on the West Coast, that caught my attention.

Venice, a beachfront neighborhood of Los Angeles, has been called Union Square, New York, on steroids. Both Union Square and Venice are packed with street vendors and musicians, Krishna followers and break-dancers. During the early twentieth century it was considered the Coney Island of the Pacific. An extended visit is not necessary to understand why that label stuck.

Gondolas cruise canals lined with palm trees, which seem straight out of that other Venice halfway around the world. Perhaps they are more like something you would find in Disneyland, only forty miles to the east.

There is an old-fashioned boardwalk populated by snake charmers and fortune-tellers, mimes and musicians, jugglers and tarot card readers. There is the weight lifting mecca of Muscle Beach. There is also a greater concentration of artists, eccentrics, and bohemians than in any other venue in Los Angeles.

In the midst of the sideshow, a rabbi tends to her offbeat flock and struggles to stave off a family tragedy. Naomi Levy shares her home with husband, Rob Eshman, publisher and editor in chief of Tribe Media, a multimedia company based in L.A. Their son, Adi, and daughter, Noa, fill out the family, joined by chickens and two pet pygmy goats in the backyard—positively de rigueur in Venice Beach. When she was a child, Noa was tentatively diagnosed with ataxia-telangiectasia, or A-T, a progressive, degenerative neurological condition. The disease affects various organs in the immune and nervous systems. Invariably, A-T is fatal.

In 1984, Levy was in the first class of women to enter the rabbinical school at the Jewish Theological Seminary in New York. In 1989, she became the first female Conservative rabbi to have her own pulpit on the West Coast. She remained there until 1996, when she stepped down to have more time for writing and teaching and taking care of her two small children.

In 2004, in another unconventional move, Levy founded a Jewish community called Nashuva, which translates from the Hebrew to "we will return." Nashuva is a community that has no official membership and no dues. There is a focus on outreach to unaffiliated Jews and to those in interfaith relationships.

The growing community has a special appeal to those who have wandered away from Judaism, as well as to Jews who are deeply involved in social justice movements. Shabbat, or Sabbath services, feature rock music, African, and reggae mixed with traditional Jewish songs and prayers. Naomi adds meditation to the mix, which she says has long been a part of the Jewish tradition.

After our initial contact, I wanted to reach out to the rabbi to continue our conversation about how she had coped with her daughter's illness, but I had difficulty connecting. I grew weary of message machines. Then Naomi left a message for me, explaining that she had been out of touch because she herself was in the midst of three complicated surgeries. She sounded guarded, offering no further details. When we finally connected, the rabbi told me what had been going on during the period of radio silence.

Naomi had been diagnosed with an infiltrative basal cell tumor on her face. That wasn't as serious as the melanoma she had feared, but it still required several invasive surgeries. "They got really good margins, but they took off my nose," she said about the surgeries. Say, what? I thought.

"They had to take off other things, like parts of my forehead and my scalp. They had to create a nose for me. It looked like a freak show because my forehead was connected to my nose." Dire as this surgery sounded, Naomi seemed strangely calm about the situation.

"I am taking it one day at a time" was her only comment to me. I already felt for her, and we had not yet delved into her daughter's illness. I asked her to talk to me about Noa.

At the time of Noa's diagnosis, Naomi and Rob had known for some time that something was not quite right with her. The child's speech was slurred, and she did not walk until she was two. By the time Noa was five, she still did not walk normally. The couple was alerted by doctors that this might well be serious. "We were in the dark about it. We had no idea what it was," Naomi explained. "We went doctor to doctor, test to test. People were unsure what it was and how to deal with it."

During this period of uncertainty, Naomi encountered a woman whose twenty-year-old daughter, Rebecca, was struggling with ataxia-telangiectasia. In January 1999, the woman asked Naomi to deliver the keynote address at a fund-raiser for Rebecca. After Naomi's speech, the woman asked her to bless Rebecca before the hundreds of people who had gathered to support the young woman and her family. During the blessing, Naomi could hear many people weeping.

After the blessing, a doctor who was receiving an award for his breakthroughs in A-T research also spoke. He said that Rebecca's disease was a blessing because it had led to the funding of such important research. The statement horrified Naomi because she saw no blessing, only pain and suffering. I have met my share of doctors whose feet stay firmly in their mouths.

Noa's doctor had suspected she, too, had A-T, but the jury was still out. "I could not begin to imagine the torment Rebecca and her parents were living with daily," Levy later wrote in *Hope Will Find You*, her book about Noa's struggle for health.

"What did I believe? Did I believe in a God who could cure Rebecca? . . . [Who] would miraculously undo what nature and genes had done? No, not exactly. But I wanted to believe it. I prayed for that kind of faith in God's supernatural powers and at the same time I prayed for Rebecca's doctors. I hoped scientists could learn to correct the problem, treat the problem, cure the problem."

Two years passed. On a Friday evening in July 2001, at the start of the Sabbath, Naomi and her family were gathered for dinner when the phone rang. It was the same physician who had shocked Naomi at the fund-raiser for Rebecca. "I had a suspicion I was right about her," the doctor said of Noa. "The tests took months . . . She has A-T."

Naomi's world had shattered. "My legs crumbled beneath me," she wrote. "I was sitting on the floor. I started squeaking. Crying . . . I was pinned to the floor by a gravitational force so strong I felt like the wood beneath me was about to give way and I would be sucked into the center of hell itself."

What a way for a physician to break tragic news. The call was brief and without empathy. "I was caught off guard," Naomi remembered. She had believed no news was good news and was stunned by what the doctor said. Naomi exploded in agony. She wrote that the doctor told her, "'Most parents are so grateful when I give them the news.'" Naomi's response was swift: "'Grateful? They're GRATEFUL?' I hung up. I hung up on my daughter's doctor."

Despite what the doctor had said on the phone, the diagnosis still was considered tentative. Other physicians Naomi consulted told her they would not be able to be certain of the grim prognosis until seven more years passed, when Noa would be about thirteen. The subtext was, if she lives that long. By that age Noa would be growing stronger or weaker, and they would have their answer.

A-T is devastating. Respiratory infections and malignancies are common. The breakdown of the body is slow but steady. Once the doctor delivered his bad news, everyone in the family watched Noa closely, looking for any of the changes that had been described to them. All understood how frightening the possibilities were. So began the long family vigil.

Did you hope at that time? I asked Naomi. You are a rabbi. Did Judaism tell you how to hope? "In Jewish life, there is not a lot of dogma," she answered. "No one is checking your faith system when you come into a synagogue. No one is asking you to proclaim a certain doctrine of hope. But *hope* is a very important Jewish word. The name of Israel's national anthem is 'Hatikvah,' which means 'the hope.' The hope 'to be a free people in our own land' is two thousand years old."

Next year in Jerusalem is the phrase that ends both the Passover seder and the Yom Kippur services. That defiant and hopeful cry speaks to the Jewish longing to one day rebuild the temple that was destroyed two millennia ago and to return home. For Naomi and Rob, however, home was under siege.

Naomi clearly remembers the jumble of emotions she felt as she tried to make sense of Noa's illness, to figure out how to live with the terrible uncertainty. "I went through many different phases and, honestly, some did not make us hopeful at all. It was like a thick blackness that didn't seem to have any contours."

How did you function as a rabbi during this time? I asked. "It was a time I didn't know how to pray or what to pray for. Should I pray to God to take this away? Did I really believe God had given this to her? I couldn't believe that God would do that." The same questions she had asked when she saw Rebecca's suffering were surfacing in her own life.

The cries of *Why me? What have I done to deserve this?* are natural, if not inevitable. Even Job, the Bible's long-suffering servant of god, never lost faith.

I asked Naomi if her own faith had cracked. "My faith is a complicated thing. When I was sixteen in Brooklyn, my father was murdered. A lot of the work I did to figure out where I stand vis-à-vis God, I thought, was done. I already had fought that battle. I no longer saw God as a superman. I was not waiting for God to protect us."

Naomi had written about this earlier tragedy in her book *To Begin Again*, which tells of her journey back to believing in God after a long period of anger and darkness. The god Naomi serves, she told me, is not a god who intervenes in a direct way, changing people's lives. I knew she was thinking of Noa's struggle.

With the grim news of Noa's disease, Naomi once again had to fight her way back to the light, to a feeling of hope. Despite being a rabbi and having been through intense suffering before, there were years when she felt lost.

Naomi was angry. When I asked about that, she spoke slowly and carefully about her reaction to the prospect of losing her daughter. The anger she felt at that time was unavoidable, she said. She believes rage in the face of such a horror is natural, even inevitable, and she offers no apology.

After the diagnosis, Naomi was determined to identify any therapy that might help Noa. Naomi discovered that taking Noa on endless rounds of doctor appointments was grueling. Handling the paperwork required by her insurance company became a full-time job. She gave up her rabbinical duties.

Becoming a caregiver rather than a rabbi upended Naomi's sense of self. She had accomplished so much in her work and won acclaim as both a rabbi and writer. "And now look at me," she wrote plaintively, almost as a cry. "I had no ambition. None left. I was so tired. I didn't know where I ended and Noa began."

Yet even in the early days of her pain, Naomi was able to take refuge and find joy in the arms of her family. The love of those we hold close offers a deep reservoir of hope. I learned that from my own family during my struggles with sickness. There is an unbreakable emotional link between parents, children, and siblings. Rabbi Levy recounted how the wisdom of her children offered its own brand of solace.

"My son, Adi, who is two years older than Noa, is the only person in the world who treated Noa like just another kid. That's how he saw her. Noa was a little sister. Adi was a big brother." Adi was resolute, insisting on seeing his family as normal. "He just thought, oh, all little sisters can't walk. Just watching Noa steal a toy out of his hand, it gave me hope."

Naomi's husband, Rob, was also a strong source of support. At the time Naomi felt most lost, Rob somehow had found an inner compass and become more productive and active than ever. "I was drowning and Rob seemed to be rising," she wrote. "I wanted him to describe the world as he saw it, the world of hope."

Naomi's prayer life was in a state of turmoil, and she began leaning hard on her husband. "Rob, who had always been a skeptical Jew, began making all sorts of bargains with God," she told me. She would watch Rob in the synagogue. She said it calmed her to sit beside him when he was deep in thought.

"I wanted to know what he believed, what he was saying to God." He told Naomi, "It can't hurt to pray." She said, "Rob was praying to *Just in Case*—that was the name of his God."

Rob told Naomi he would be at work and suddenly be seized by fear. Panic over Noa's condition gripped his chest and sent his heart racing until his body was covered in sweat. But he would willfully push the fear out of his mind. Naomi asked him how he was able to do that. As she wrote in her book: "'Denial,' Rob said, 'don't underestimate it.'" Naomi says she was terrible at denial.

Naturally, I recognized his line of thinking, since I am also a student of denial. Denial has been a powerful coping mechanism during my many skirmishes with sickness. I have lived through crises and been able to survive emotionally by denying the inevitability of possible outcomes. The line between probable and a done deal is conveniently blurred.

Denial has allowed me to expand my life. Even when the

odds are stacked against me, denial allows me to keep spirits up and anxiety down. Distilled to its essence, I believe denial can be an effective strategy for fostering hope.

Gradually, Naomi began focusing on the good in her life. She traveled to Boston to visit her mother, always a source of strength for her. The night Naomi fell apart after hearing Noa's diagnosis, her mother had found just the right words to say to her, as she recounted in *Hope Will Find You*: "'How can a doctor who calls with bad results during Shabbat dinner possibly know anything?'"

After the trip to Boston, Naomi wrote, "I could see something was beginning to shift inside me. Yes, Noa was still struggling. Yes, [Noa's ordeal] was all so unfair. Yes, there was that question mark hanging over our heads. But I was beginning to see the blessings of the moment."

Naomi seemed to have developed a new strategy for finding her feet. It was not clear if this was her way of preparing for the worst or of making the best of the bad hand they had been dealt. I did not have the heart to ask what those blessings were.

What Naomi did say about this inner shift was that she had discovered an important lesson in her life: "You can't live your life wishing things were different from what they are. The truth is, things were ambiguous and scary and they were also wonderful."

"How were they wonderful?" I asked.

"I have a husband who is my soul mate," she said to me. "We have two incredible children and an adorable dog who is always destroying things." I get it. I travel that road. Those are reasons for gratitude, important ingredients in the life of a family.

"I was a lot of things at once. At the same time, I was just a mother playing with her kids. It was not just one tone, one color. For that I am grateful. I didn't have the luxury of not being a mother to my children. Both of them were my salvation."

For those of us blessed with kids, I believe doing well by them and guiding them toward a meaningful life are the noblest of all pursuits. Making money and winning promotions, collecting awards or accruing power, somehow seem empty compared to raising our children to be good people. Our other job is to protect them from harm at all costs. That was something Naomi felt powerless to do. Her fears for Noa sometimes overwhelmed her.

In her effort to control her level of fear, Naomi experimented with Buddhism. A few years after Noa's diagnosis, Naomi began attending meditation sessions. One day, the instructor told the class she would teach them the death meditation. The central message was that death can come at any minute for anyone.

The meditation did not comfort Naomi. It terrified her. Then she thought of the teachings of a legendary Hasidic master, Rabbi Nachman of Breslov. Rabbi Nachman told his followers life is brief and perilous, and we therefore must live it without fear. Fear can paralyze a person. Naomi began to see that the awareness of death did not cast a shadow over life; instead, it was a route to living a fuller life.

"This teaching became my mantra when I was worrying over Noa and the death sentence the doctor had put on her," Naomi wrote to me. "I could feel the power of the death meditation working through me. I was becoming more aware of how little time I had left, and I felt a new courage to try things I had never tried before."

As time passed, something inside Naomi continued to stir. She was realizing how durable and resilient Noa herself had become. The child was blessed in many ways, calm and wise in the face of her illness. Rob called her his Zen master. As Noa struggled with a failing body, her spirits seemed to soar.

Naomi told me about a morning when Noa was having problems with balance and walking. Naomi said it would be okay for her to stay home from school, but Noa made it clear she wanted to go. If she could just pray, she said, she would be okay. Naomi watched Noa singing her morning prayers in Hebrew.

"She was just praying from joy," Naomi told me. "I could see how prayer would give her the strength to pick her body up. Prayer would give her the strength to walk. You just forget how much something as simple as a prayer can say to you."

This was a scene Naomi included in her book. "A serenity started to flow through her body . . . Her mood changed, her posture changed, her expression changed. When she was done singing, she walked straight up to me with strength and steadiness and said, 'I'm ready for school now.' And she was." Naomi read this episode in her daughter's life as Noa's hope reborn, and she took comfort from it.

After the seven-year waiting period doctors required before they could make a definitive diagnosis of A-T, Naomi and Rob saw that Noa was growing stronger. If she really did have A-T, the disease would have ravaged her body by then. Noa's neurologist had been telling the family for some time that she did not present as a typical A-T child. The doctor believed Noa had a static condition she would continue to live with, though he had no name for it.

Noa's death sentence had quietly been lifted. Shaking off the dreaded letters, *A-T*, was the end of the treacherous journey. Life gradually changed. It was as if Noa had clenched her teeth, tightened her muscles, and pulled herself up and out of the deep hole. There was no high drama, no moment of claiming victory. There only was immense relief.

As Noa neared her thirteenth birthday, it came time to prepare her for her bat mitzvah. Studying for the ceremony began many months in advance, and Naomi was uncertain that Noa would be able to master the complicated Hebrew required. However, Noa learned so rapidly that Naomi was astounded. She was taken with the emotional depth of Noa's understanding of the portion of the Old Testament she had to read.

The passage was from the Book of Isaiah. Fittingly, the words were about hope. When Naomi asked her daughter what the reading meant to her, Noa answered in words from the passage that gave Naomi's book its title. "'Maybe God is telling us that if you don't like your life, if you really try to enjoy your life, you will find hope. No . . . hope will find you.'"

That is a powerful belief, and perhaps a message to all who are sick. For Naomi, it was a reminder of Psalm 23, of the line that reads, "Surely goodness and mercy shall follow me all the days of my life, and I shall dwell in the house of the lord forever." As Naomi wrote in her book, "Goodness and mercy are stalking you. That is what Noa was saying."

Noa and Naomi had traded roles. Who was the parent, and who the child? Who the teacher, and who the student? That no longer was clear. "There is no question," Naomi told me. "Noa raised me." They had come full circle.

CHAPTER 10

Invading the Vatican

n April 2013, I stared out the small window of our mammoth airplane, eyeing the fuel truck on the tarmac as workmen pumped high-grade kerosene into the tanks under the wings. Soon our lives would be in the hands of these and other airline workers, many of who were milling about and checking the jet as I watched. Flying anywhere at forty thousand feet is a giant leap of faith.

So, too, was our expedition to the Vatican. We would be trying to understand the highly complex, evolving landscape of modern medicine. We were going to probe the promise of stem cell therapies. Meredith told me she was full of hope. I felt buoyed by the energy coming from her. I was no longer experiencing wild excitement, but rather a quiet confidence that I was on the verge of something good happening.

There was no question in my mind that I was losing my deadly duel with disease. Why not give in to the temptation to hope? We were about to be presented with new possibility. Scientists, working toward saving the sick with stem cells would take center stage. This colloquy would mean listening and learning from them, as well as sharing my own experiences. I knew I would benefit from their presentations. As much as I hated to admit it, I was in the market for a miracle. I was searching for the magic bullet that had eluded my doctors so far. Perhaps the Vatican would help me find it.

I still could not get used to the idea that I would be speaking at the Vatican. As we flew east, I felt a twinge of emotion. I thought of my Irish Catholic grandparents long gone. They would have been thrilled that I was giving a speech to a meeting at the seat of their religion.

I would be approaching the Vatican with a smile and a receptive mind. Every pore on my body was wide open, especially when it came to subjects of science and the upcoming symposium. We had been assured by Robin Smith that advances in combating disease would be the primary focus at the conference. I trusted Robin and believed her when she said that the Church's commitment to medical research was strong.

Though I felt well prepared, it was not completely clear what was expected of me at the conference, and I was distracted by personal possibilities. I wanted to store my fantasies away but was having trouble actually doing that. Deep inside, something was still stirring. It was soft and subtle, but I could not get past the chance that something could change my life as a result of these meetings. This was my shot.

Meredith fell asleep shortly after takeoff and awakened somewhere over the Atlantic. I asked her if she thought I was desperate and confused. "Maybe," was her only answer. Thank you for that, I softly said as she closed her eyes again. It was time for me to stop killing myself with questions. But I could not sleep. My obsession with finding help had a childlike quality, and I felt quietly self-conscious.

I decided to turn my attention to the prospect of seeing our children in Rome. In two days, all three, grown and launched in their own lives, would be converging on that magic city, Ben from China, where he was working in the nuclear power industry, and Gabe and Lily from Chicago. Rome would be an exciting venue for us to have a family reunion. It would also be their first time speaking publicly about the impact of their father's MS on their own lives. They would be addressing a sold-out luncheon at the Vatican. I don't believe I ever did that at their age.

The truth is, my kids have always been smarter and exponentially more sophisticated than I was at their young ages. They had launched and gone into their respective orbits. I have spent substantial time worrying about the health of all three and knew that would not end for many decades. Parents want to keep protecting kids, but that race has been run. I know these young people will find success. I desperately want sound health to be part of the package.

We made our way through the concourse of Leonardo da Vinci airport, grateful to be off the airplane and in Rome. We spotted the representatives from the Stem for Life Foundation who had come to pick us up. They herded us, along with a number of others who were part of the conference, into cars and vans that would take us to our hotels. Drivers on the congested roads leaned on horns and cut their cars and trucks across heavy traffic as we neared the center of the city. Exhaust fumes filled the air and our lungs. This was the Rome I remembered well.

From a distance we caught a glimpse of the Papal Palace, home to the Sistine Chapel, where God and man reach out to touch fingertips. Michelangelo painted the ceiling of the Sistine Chapel in the early sixteenth century. To me, there is no greater symbol of Christianity.

The van delivered us to a classic old hotel on the Via Veneto. After checking in and unpacking, we met Robin and her fiancé, Matthew, for dinner. The plan was to talk through my presentation one last time, but the wine got in the way. Maybe that was just as well. I was unnerved whenever I thought too much about my role in the conference.

The next day Meredith and I would have some precious time to relax until evening, when we would be attending a small private dinner at the Vatican. There we would break bread with a select group of conference participants, though we weren't sure who. Until then, our time was our own.

Rome has special significance for Meredith and me. We had spent time there after we were married and roamed the streets for days. My hope was to relive those wonderful times. We intended to walk the ancient city, visiting the Spanish Steps and the Villa Borghese, which held great memories.

As we left the hotel the next morning, my feet had barely touched the ground when my bubble burst. I was unable to negotiate the cobblestone streets or walk more than a block or two. What could I have been thinking? I was stunned by my pipe dream. My idea of dancing through the city with Meredith had been my private movie, and it was already over. My denial was as out of control as my health.

After we returned from Rome, my sister saw a photo of me standing in front of the Colosseum. "What do you know," she wrote in an email, "a wreck in front of a ruin." The quip pretty much captured my own view of myself. I saw a train wreck in the mirror every morning. "Other people don't see you that way," Meredith regularly reminded me. "You used to worry yourself to death about how the kids saw you," she would say. "You could not get used to the fact that they would roll the ball back to you after your throw to them. They understood you couldn't see."

Meredith paused. "Listen, Jack, do you really think they thought less of you because of that?" I had no answer. I did not know Jack, but Meredith certainly sounded contemptuous when she spoke his name. Meredith was right. I knew how hard I could be on myself, as if I were at fault for being sick. I could not break that pattern.

Returning to the hotel after my failed attempt at a walk, I saw the lobby was bulging with serious-sounding individuals, many of who seemed to know one another. They were talking in small groups. I felt out of my element, surrounded by world-class scientists and physicians. But I knew I had something that fascinated them—my life story.

That story was compelling. I was a body in motion now, a man on a mission. I was tired of playing victim. I was determined to be part of a solution. And I was a body out of control, in need of help. What was at stake for me in the race to find effective stem cell therapies would be evident to anyone who saw me struggle and strain to walk. I would be the lead-off hitter at the conference—a very unsteady one, but I was suited up and ready.

Our kids were due into Rome soon. These young people were forced to grow up fast, never knowing if there was a target on their backs. At this event, they might be expected to put fear for their futures on display. We did not know how comfortable they would be, talking about a matter as personal as illness in the family. That they would be doing this at the Vatican had to be daunting. They, too, were bringing a sense of mission with them.

Our kids are old beyond their years. They have seen a lot. They have watched me fall and struggle to my feet numerous times. Each had read my books and watched Meredith and me on television, talking about coping with serious sickness.

What goes on in the heads of those kids may forever remain a mystery. Personal fears are kept private. How much they would reveal in an intimidating public place I had no idea.

I did know that when I discussed the conference with them over the phone, they seemed ready, with no apparent qualms. We would be seeing them soon. But first there was that dinner at the Vatican to attend. At the appointed time, Meredith and I went down to the lobby, where we were to meet our fellow guests and be directed to one of the cars that would transport us to the Holy See.

The Vatican is a mysterious city within a city. As we approached the fortress, we could see the Swiss Guards silently standing on the cobbled street at the gate. Their berets were perched jauntily on their heads, the billowy pants of their distinctive striped uniforms puffing slightly in the breeze. The guards seemed frozen in time.

Though these Swiss Catholics once bore swords—at one time, even priests were armed—they now patrol unarmed. The men waved our modest motorcade through the gates, and almost at once we found ourselves deeper into the immaculately manicured Vatican grounds than most tourists are allowed to venture.

The animated conversation that had filled the car gradually tapered and turned into silence. As we drove slowly along the ancient roads that wound through the Vatican grounds, looking out on the wide, perfectly manicured lawns, everyone seemed subdued. We retreated into ourselves. It was hard not to be awestruck by what we were seeing, as we seemed to travel back in time.

Our cars came to a stop at the ancient structure in the heart of the Vatican Gardens where the Pontifical Academy of Sciences is located. The origins of the academy date back to Rome in 1603. The building where it is headquartered, the Casina Pio IV, is even older, having been completed in 1561 as a summer residence for Pope Pius IV.

Waiting outside to greet us was a group of Vatican officials, including Cardinal Gianfranco Ravasi, who was easy to spot from a distance, his bright red skullcap and cummerbund a welcoming beacon. Cardinal Ravasi serves in the Roman Curia, the pope's inner circle, and is president of the Pontifical Council for Culture, which was hosting the conference.

Another of the priests who had come to receive us was a young Polish monsignor, Tomasz Trafny, who told us in clear English to call him Tommy. Tommy moved with ease among both his older colleagues and the guests. Everyone in the welcoming party was well prepared. Each priest and Vatican official who approached us knew our names and enough about us to make sense of our roles at the conference. When Tommy got to me, he introduced the subject of multiple sclerosis and mentioned my books, with which he seemed to be familiar.

The dinner had a surprisingly easygoing air of informality and candor. Tommy told us about once being engaged to be married at home in Poland. Even as wedding presents were arriving, Tommy said, he could hear the calling to the priesthood. Tommy would don the white collar, and his fiancé, a nun's habit.

Tommy was a player. He was director of the Vatican's newly formed Science and Faith Foundation. He had given an interview to CNN on the occasion of the stem cell conference in which he acknowledged, "There was a time when theologians thought they understood everything, but we learned the lesson from history. If you look at what is going on today, you will see that theologians are very careful about what they are thinking or speaking about related to scientific issues."

Tommy impressed everyone with the seriousness of his commitment to scientific inquiry. He patiently explained that researchers from around the world were routinely invited to meetings at the Vatican to present their work without regard to religion or nationality. I did not know that. Even my mother would have approved.

There seemed to be no agenda for the evening, other than to put us at ease and allow us to get to know one another. Our disparate group included several scientists and researchers, as well as a prominent columnist, a billionaire philanthropist, and a physician entrepreneur. Many—if not most—of us were not Catholic. All approached the issues at hand from different angles and with varied expectations. Clearly, the conference would have nothing to do with religion.

Given the Vatican's long, dark history of persecuting scientists whose findings were deemed heretical, I had associated the place with hard-edged orthodoxy. But if the Vatican seemed an unlikely venue to pursue questions of science, it was also true that, just as Robin had told us, the institution now seemed determined to value pure science.

Pope Francis was new on the job. We did not know if we would meet him. Francis had received a degree as a chemical technician before entering the priesthood. Years later he would endorse climate change science. This was a new era in the Catholic Church. The Church still opposed using embryonic stem cells for medical research, but once scientists decided adult stem cells could be more effective in disease treatment, the Church bought in. There was a new truce between the Church and secular science.

Physicians and researchers are increasingly using autologous stem cells in their work. Autologous cells are a patient's own. Because they come from the patient's body, these cells minimize both the risk of complications and rejection. So they serve science as well as patients. The Vatican was eager to move beyond old controversies and wasted no time setting up scientific meetings on this revolutionary advance. Such gatherings might put the past to rest and speed up the future.

For my own reasons I was ready and eager to play ball. On

the opening day of the conference, I got to know a few more of the players on the new scorecard. As attendees from around the world milled about and talked in small groups before the proceedings began, I spoke with my old acquaintance and fellow panelist Dr. Saud Sadiq.

I had eavesdropped as Dr. Sadiq stood in a hall and described his work to others. I don't speak science and could not parse too much of what he was saying. Dr. Sadiq's research was in an early phase of inquiry. That much was clear. I learned that he was intimately involved with some kind of cell research, although I did not know if he was actually treating patients.

As we chatted, we were standing directly in front of the tiered amphitheater where scientists would soon be presenting their work. Although priceless religious art, paintings, tapestries, and sculpture seemed to fill every square inch of the hallways and rooms of all the other buildings in the Vatican, the large space that housed the amphitheater was austere. The surroundings bore no trace of any religion and were empty of the lavish art and artifacts I associated with the sprawling grounds. The space felt cold, even sterile.

I figured that by offering a deeply personal account of living with a serious autoimmune condition, I was supposed to provide some much-needed warmth. I planned to humanize illness before the scientists got around to the impersonal discussion of how to treat the bodies in the beds.

I had prepared, but I hadn't actually written anything for my presentation. That was unbridled chutzpah, perhaps, but my failing vision would not allow me to read a speech anyway, even if I rested my forehead on the page. And describing the patient experience of dealing with MS would not present much of a challenge for me. I lived it every day. I had coexisted with the crippling condition for more than four decades.

In giving talks, I have learned to think through what I want to say and then wing it. I want to speak from the heart. It's a high-wire act with no net, but audiences appreciate the eye contact. To connect can be to communicate.

As the time for the session came, people took their seats in the amphitheater and talk subsided to whispers, then ceased. I had approached the day with surprising calm. When I noted the utter silence in the large space, however, I was jolted by a measure of self-doubt. I took a breath and forged ahead. People were there to listen and learn. I believed I had something to say worth hearing.

Meredith and I were seated facing the audience. Archbishop Ravasi sat behind us, Tommy next to him. The cardinal was up first, speaking in Italian and reading from a script to welcome the attendees. Robin spoke next, introducing Meredith, who would be acting as the host for the day's business.

Robin cited Meredith's credentials as a journalist and her work as an advocate for those living with MS. "Then there's

Meredith's passion to help anyone suffering from chronic disease," Robin said, "especially those living with multiple sclerosis. Meredith has been a tireless advocate for the disease, and cell therapies do hold the promise of a cure."

The promise of a cure? That is swinging for the fences, I thought. Waiting for a cure would be like holding out for a miracle. All I could bring myself to hope for was some relief from my symptoms. The idea of putting down the cane or seeing more clearly seemed unrealistic. Robin was thinking big.

Meredith began, "I'm not just a journalist here looking for answers. More importantly, I'm a wife looking for hope. My husband, Richard Cohen, was diagnosed with multiple sclerosis when he was twenty-five." Meredith's voice cracked with emotion. "I met him a few years later. Despite the fact that Richard was kind of a jerk, I fell in love with him." Meredith had a wonderful sense of the moment and knew how to calm herself. "We got married and had three wonderful kids, and I soon discovered that chronic illness is truly a family affair." Meredith was in control, subtly setting up the theme of the family luncheon that would follow the session.

She introduced me to the still-silent audience. "He covered wars in Central America and the Middle East," she said, teeing up my talk with drama, "even though he is legally blind, which didn't make it easy to dodge bullets." She concluded her remarks, and I got up to speak. By now the silence seemed deafening. I wondered if the audience could hear me think. Cardinal Ravasi in his opening comments had mentioned words that he thought were important in the pursuit of cures. *Culture* and *faith* and even *love* were among them. In my talk, I referred to his remarks, suggesting there was an additional word missing: *hope*.

"This morning I want to emphasize the importance of hope. Hope is elusive. Hope is difficult to grasp, more difficult even to hold close. Hope is very hard to sustain." No one knows this better than I do. "When I was diagnosed, forty years ago, there was no hope," I continued. "My neurologist told me I had MS. He said, 'I'm sorry' and never talked about another appointment. He never discussed a strategy, a plan, because there was none. There were no therapies. Times have changed," I said, leaving out the nagging thought that the more things change, the more they stay the same.

I went on to describe the psychological beating patients take. "It is hard to get up every day and look in the mirror. We are not the people we used to be, in terms of what we do and who we are. The assault is not just on our bodies; it's on our spirit, on how we see ourselves, our self-esteem, our self-confidence, our willingness to go out and try to have a future." My building emotion took me by surprise. I usually keep my feelings in check, especially in public.

I recounted my recent decision to quit the regular trips to the neurologist. I felt I had been relying on therapies that did little or nothing for me. This was Band-Aid medicine, applied to a wound that was festering. I looked into the amphitheater and saw heads nodding. Presentations were simultaneously translated into six languages. Some in the audience had headphones on. I wondered if they were listening to music.

I ended the talk by speaking of my optimism about the potential for stem cell therapies. "I look at MS and the work being done with adult stem cell therapy and it is extraordinary. I believe that in the future, patients like me will all be seeking these therapies." That sounded lofty, but I was only pleading for help.

The enthusiastic response was gratifying. The applause felt good, and afterward a number of people approached me, eager to share their own personal stories. This was unusual because scientific gatherings do not usually generate emotion. All I wanted, really, was the confidence and credibility to walk up to any of the scientists in the large room and ask, "What can you do for me?"

It was clear from the buzz that cell therapy was currently under way around the world. This was not some future plan. If I could connect with the right persons, there would be a lot to discuss. A lot was happening in other countries, which meant procedures would not be regulated the same way as they were in the United States. I was ready to travel anywhere in the world, on foot if necessary. I did wonder about the safety of procedures done overseas though.

Dr. Sadiq spoke next. The man got right to the point, as if reading my mind. He described where he saw science and medicine at that time. In his talk he made it clear that he was already hard at work treating patients with some form of cell therapy. I would later learn he was experimenting with different kinds of cells from adults.

Sadiq also was very human, expressing feelings that I had not observed in many of the doctors I had seen over the years. "You've just heard from Richard how patients can start to lose hope," the doctor said. "And as physicians, I might add, we also find moments of darkness, moments when we tend to lose hope as we see patients like Richard."

I was seated at an angle where eye contact was impossible. I wondered if Sadiq could feel me reaching out to him. I felt sheepishly like a New Age supplicant trying out a form of psychic communication. I sensed a connection. My epiphany was almost jarring when I realized I had to make a meeting with Sadiq happen back in New York.

"We often turn to our faith and to the work of our fellow scientists to find inspiration," Dr. Sadiq continued. "But our greatest hope and our greatest inspiration usually comes from our patients. I dedicate this talk to all my patients who suffer with multiple sclerosis, for the inspiration and hope that they have given me."

I was accustomed to the arrogance of many physicians. This man seemed to be different. Dr. Sadiq's humility and empathy stood out. Dr. Sadiq and Dr. Burt had been seen arguing loudly in the corridor before the session that morning. I heard about it later and had no idea what the disagreement was. Sadiq did not seem like the shouting type. His manner seemed gentle. Although there was controversy about Sadiq's work among his fellow neurologists, he was fiercely loved by his patients. His devotion to them was legendary.

A dark-skinned Muslim in a white world, Sadiq wore his credentials as an outsider proudly. The man was a maverick who bucked the establishment. He was my kind of guy.

When the morning session ended, I realized that the Vatican had been transformed into a medical marketplace. Business was getting done in hallways, as scientists traded information about research and clinical trials. Hello, I silently yelled. Let me in. No one was selling, but I was eager to buy.

A palpable energy filled this place. I could not shake off that twinge of hope. I realized that, at the very least, I wanted to hope. That desire was fed by our kids' presence in Rome. If any of them were to develop MS, I wanted an effective therapy in place and available, even if it was too late for me.

Meredith and I were about to join the star attractions, Ben, Gab, and Lily, at the luncheon. The event was sponsored by Opexa Therapeutics, a Texas pharmaceutical company that was in the middle of a clinical trial, testing B cell therapy. This unproved treatment targets specific immune cells that may be partially responsible for MS misery. We were friendly with Neil Warma, the Opexa CEO who would be moderating the discussion. Still, we were apprehensive, watching our kids go public about what had been mostly unspoken as they grew up. The conversation would be carried on closed-circuit television throughout the Vatican for the other conferees as they ate their lunches. B cell therapy is freaking complicated and not part of our story. Neil is.

The first questioner asked how much MS dominates our lives. Meredith told the audience there is more to us than multiple sclerosis. "On a good day, it's not a topic of conversation. It really isn't. You just sort of live your life. On a bad day, it's that elephant that's always in the room." All three kids nodded.

Gabe jumped in, agreeing. "It really becomes part of who we are, part of our family. It's something we just live with." Lily followed suit: "Overall, it's something that's there, and it's not above everything else." There was a moment of silence. The three of them seemed relaxed and ready to share.

Lily then offered a thought about the importance of perspective. "You both raised us very much in a great way, with this sort of attitude that you shouldn't sweat the small things and you shouldn't let the stupid things upset you." She paused. "And you shouldn't let yourself be held back by illness or by any other issue like that."

Ben talked about his feelings on the possibility of being hit by MS, and he struck a defiant tone as he seconded Lily's admonition not to allow it to hold him back. "I think that humor is a very important thing," he said. "Damned if [the fear of] MS is going to stop me from what doing what I want to do. That was certainly true of my grandfather, and it is certainly true of my dad."

I admired the defiance. Once again, I knew I would do anything I could to spare my children the pain of eroding health, but these young people seemed disinclined to roll over and play dead.

Ben pushed away the idea that we are different from other families. "We're normal. There's no other way to say this. We're normal. Every family has stuff they deal with." I was proud of him. I wish my Old Man had been there.

I was moved as they spoke about how MS had sculpted their worlds and how they had learned to reach beyond the illness. I was taken by their strength, which struck me as a solid foundation for hope. Meredith and I had not used the word *hope* with our children when they were young, though we did urge them to be upbeat and optimistic and certainly tried to teach them by example.

After the luncheon, the kids reverted to their young selves. They seemed not at all flustered by their performance on Vatican television. The Cohen condition was built into their lives. They had more pressing concerns, such as how they could locate some wine and where we were going for dinner. I kept quiet about how impressed I was. It did occur to me that maybe we had done something right raising them.

That night, the conference participants were offered a tour of the treasures of the Vatican. The Vatican is a maze of endless corridors that culminate in the Sistine Chapel. The walk to the Chapel, a long trek through a rich history documented by some of the world's greatest artists and craftsmen, was exhausting. I had declined the offer of a wheelchair, but changed my mind long before the evening ended. That was just another concession to the beast inside me.

In the days that followed, I met scientists involved in the earliest stem cell therapies for a wide range of diseases, including cancers and diabetes and neurodegenerative conditions such as Parkinson's and Alzheimer's. MS joins the roster of cruel conditions scientists hope to treat with stem cells. For those of us with secondary progressive MS, life can be particularly frustrating because there have never been any conventional treatments for our form of the disease. People with SPMS are orphans in MS world.

Doctors focus on the illnesses scientists believe offer the best chance of finding treatments or cures. They go for the low-hanging fruit. I had figured my type of MS was something they would tackle only after they'd had more success with other forms of the disease. That is not what I was hearing at the Vatican.

It was not just research that dominated conversation. Real

people in many places were being treated at that moment. Procedures were being developed and dispensed *now*. Scientists were speaking in the present tense. So were many of the business interests that owned the well-funded companies that were finding applications for the research. The possibilities offered in this brave new world of science were stunning.

At the Vatican, I reconnected with an old colleague and friend who had also become interested in the potential of stem cell therapy. Allen Pizzey, with whom I had worked at CBS News, stopped in for a visit. Pizzey lived in Rome and was the network's point man at the Vatican, when he was not covering wars in every hellhole on earth. He had lived in Rome since 1989. Our paths had crossed in various parts of the world.

Allen and I took a short walk on the Vatican grounds. I noticed he was staring down toward his feet, a survival strategy I had adopted long ago. Allen told me in even tones that he had been diagnosed with retinitis pigmentosa and was slowly losing his vision. Allen had been in combat zones for decades. Now he was fighting to save his eyesight. He was looking into the possibility of joining a stem cell clinical trial in California. "I believe stem cells might be the answer," he later wrote in an email. "Without that hope you might as well slit your wrists."

I admired Pizzey. I noted the same calm during our conversation he had demonstrated under fire in our work. There was no hint of drama in his narrative. His commitment to covering the world seemed to outstrip his concern for covering his own ass. I wondered if this was denial or a dedication to journalism.

As the conference drew to a close, it was nearing time to reenter my world. I needed to think realistically about all the blue-sky therapies in my head. I thought of friends and colleagues I had lost to diseases—my old boss on the Cronkite broadcast, dead of melanoma; the newswriter for Cronkite and Rather who had recently died of gastric cancer; Ed Bradley of *60 Minutes*, taken from us by leukemia. I wondered if any of them might have been saved by one of these revolutionary treatments.

And there were the five good people profiled in my second book, *Strong at the Broken Places*. One young man was taken by muscular dystrophy. Could the others be helped? As Kurt Vonnegut wrote of Billy Pilgrim in *Slaughterhouse-Five*, I was "unstuck in time," reaching deep into the past, even as I projected into the future. I thought about these friends and colleagues on occasion, wishing I could buy them a drink.

After the final session, I asked Robin what she thought about the conference. "I thought it was a success," she said without hesitation. "I think we did a great job of exploring what is on the horizon." Then she paused. "There are more than thirty thousand trials right now. I think we are learning much more about what happens naturally in our bodies and how we can enhance it to fight whatever is happening to us."

Then do you think there is reason to hold on to hope because of this work? I asked. "A hundred percent," Robin responded. "I think we have to hold on to hope. And when we see a trial that does not work, we have to keep hoping, because we are closer than we have ever been before to something that will work."

As we left the session to return to our hotel and pack, I caught sight of Dr. Sadiq. He and his wife were in a crowd of conference-goers who were saying their goodbyes and posing for photos. The doctor and I made eye contact and worked our way over to each other. I was happy for one more chance.

We shook hands warmly and introduced our wives. I told Sadiq that I had learned a lot and was very interested in knowing more about what he was doing with stem cells. He paused for a moment and smiled. I was struck by an unfamiliar intensity in his face. The word *mystical* came to mind.

"When we get back to New York," he said, "come see me."

CHAPTER 11

Joining the Jesuits

My time at the Vatican had made me think about the Catholic Church differently. I wanted to identify a Catholic cleric with credibility as a freethinker, though I feared doctrine and dogma would get in the way. I had met Jesuits in the anti–Vietnam War movement, clergy who staked out positions on the front lines of resistance. In those years, religion met the counterculture and minds opened wide. Those priests were pretty cool and routinely bucked authority. I knew I needed to connect to a community of Jesuits.

Jesuits are a Roman Catholic order whose mission includes promoting education and charity. By reputation, Jesuits provide the intellectual backbone to Catholicism. I knew I was on target. I really wanted to hear a Catholic take on the idea of hope through the eyes of a Jesuit. Would hope float through the heavens or be nailed to old-fashioned orthodoxy? I had no clue.

Bob Doucette is an alumnus of Le Moyne College, a Jesuit school in Syracuse, New York, and sits on the Board of Regents there. He and his wife, Katie, are lifelong Catholics who seem to wander in and out of their faith. The Doucettes have been close friends of mine for many decades. They told me years ago that they invented their own brand of Catholicism, picking and choosing what beliefs make sense to them. I figured Bob would know the kind of person I was looking for. He offered to set me up with Jesuit brothers at Le Moyne.

The president of Le Moyne is the first laywoman to serve in that position at a Jesuit institution. And the college has a history of welcoming rebels. Father Daniel Berrigan, an icon of the anti–Vietnam War movement, taught there from 1957 to 1963. I could relate to his brand of faith. "Faith is rarely where your head is at," he once said, "nor is it where your heart is at. Faith is where your ass is at." Father Berrigan walked the walk, standing up and even going to prison for what he believed. Father Berrigan built a bridge even to the godless. I admired Father Berrigan, which reinforced my plan to visit Le Moyne.

When I arrived at the college, I went directly to the priests' residence, where I was greeted by Reverend David McCallum, who was waiting for me outside. Rev. McCallum is vice president for mission integration and development at Le Moyne. A tall, youthful man wearing street clothes on that hot day, the priest became David to me at our first handshake. He was truly welcoming.

Rev. George Coyne, another Jesuit with an air of informality, soon joined us. George is a retired astronomer who had been director of the Vatican Observatory in Rome for twenty-eight years, until 2006. The Vatican Observatory (Specola Vaticana) is headquartered in Castel Gandolfo, the pope's summer residence south of Rome.

George had the look of a windblown uncle, dressed in old, comfortable Saturday clothes. Meeting priests out of uniform instantly humanizes them. The starched white collars make them authority figures. Without those collars, they seemed more accessible. I felt immediately at ease.

We chatted standing still. Nobody was in a hurry to move. Standing motionless in one place is among my tougher physical challenges. When my legs began to shake, I wondered if the others noticed. Fortunately, we soon moved into the priests' residence and went to a sitting room to talk.

I wanted to start the conversation with George. I was intrigued by his story. There had been a report in the *Daily Mail* in 2006 that he had been "sacked" by Pope Benedict regarding differences over theories of evolution. Reportedly, George had dismissed intelligent design as a ruling principle and was fired because of it. George laughed off the story about his departure when I brought it up. He said it had just been time to retire.

Sacked or not, George clearly is an intellectually rigorous man and a highly respected scientist, whose beliefs might have appeared dangerous to an entrenched institution such as the Vatican. I thought he would be the perfect person to ask about pressure in the church to adhere to doctrine. From there we could move to a discussion of hope and faith.

To varying degrees, I began, the religions of the world are doctrinal. Am I wrong to assume that Catholicism is right up there with the most rigorous in terms of doctrinal demands? I asked. As he responded, George made it clear that his connection to God had primacy over all else.

"The first thing about my relationship with God is not my relationship to the Church," George said slowly and forcefully. "With faith, it seems to me, we all walk our own walks. I accept the small doctrinal content that goes with my faith . . . [but] doctrine is very secondary and minimal. Very few doctrines to which I adhere have meaning in my life." I tend to agree with him. I sprint away from all doctrines. I do not appreciate being told what to think.

Jesuits seem to bathe in abstract ideas, as if life is one long intellectual exercise. "We are less adherent to doctrine than most Catholics," George added. "I am not alone here. Certainly I share it with my Jesuit brothers." He paused, then continued. "The Catholic Church is not monolithic."

For a few hours, David and George answered my questions without hesitation. These gentlemen seemed comfortable in their skin. They are walking their own walks, as George put it, practicing their personal approach to Catholicism. That said, they do buy into the bedrock beliefs of their faith.

"I believe in the virgin birth of Jesus," George told me, as David nodded in agreement. "Although that defies knowledge, it has priority over scientific knowledge." This jolted me, but I reminded myself that I was writing a book about hope, not judging the religions of the world. If that core belief required a leap of faith, perhaps that was similar to the long jump required by hope.

Eventually David, George, and I wandered into the conversation about hope I wanted to initiate. I had to understand if their ideas about hope were only those sent down from above. Had they shaped their own feelings about hope?

David compared hope to human cells: "There is the hope, like your autoimmune cells, that is self-regenerative by some gift within us. It is the hope beyond hope that Jesus describes in the Gospels. Even in the face of what seems like the end, we are going to keep moving forward."

For those of us who struggle to stay on our feet, continuing to put one foot in front of the other, hope has special meaning. In our darkest moments, when outcomes look bleak, it can seem as if hope is all we have. We may not be brimming with hope, but surely we would be driving on empty without what little we have. The danger is when we expect hope to become a self-fulfilling prophecy. I believe having expectations sets one up for disappointment. David spoke to that concern.

"One distinction that I like to make is between hope and expectation," he said. "For me, hope is open-ended and free of any entitlement, whereas expectation puts me and my desires or sense of entitlement at the center of reality. That is a sure setup for disappointment. By contrast, hope for me is a kind of disposition of humility, gratefulness, and trust."

David and George truly seemed to have a pastoral component to their reasoning. I had the feeling they trafficked far less in religious absolutes than in spiritual guidance. They spoke softly. Hushed tones seem to be common in the Jesuit world. Soft voices often sound louder than shouts. Decades in the news business had suggested that shouting was the standard means of communication. With these gentlemen, even I became quieter, waiting to hear what else they would say.

"Hope has an end, a destination," George mused. "What is it? Is it healing? What is the object of hope?" A slight shrug punctuated the question. These were Socratic questions, and I did not think any answer was expected. Yet I had traveled to Syracuse for answers.

When I pushed, George said, "Your search for answers and not more questions is, to my mind, a treacherous path to take in one's journey in life. Hope is intimately involved in the persistent questioning that all of us have. And it is persistent." I took that to mean there really are no answers. Maybe the wisdom is in the question. Fair enough.

Still, the question George raised about the object of hope is a compelling one. Thomas Merton, a Catholic writer and Trappist monk, had warned of the perils of hoping for anything specific: "Do not depend on the hope of results . . . You may have to face the fact that your work will be apparently worthless and even achieve no result at all, if not perhaps results opposite to what you expect."

That was not a ringing endorsement of hope. But deep thinkers tend not to indulge in easy pieties. Kate Hennessy, the granddaughter of Dorothy Day, one of the cofounders of the Catholic Worker Movement, quotes Day as saying, "There are always answers. They're just not calculated to soothe."

Unlike clergy who want to offer certainty to members of their flock, the Jesuit brothers embrace big questions and contradictions. They see hope as a journey, one built on an element of mystery, which they celebrate rather than greet with agony. These men have a highly evolved tolerance for ambiguity.

In the end, however, both men seem to believe hope must be linked to faith. George said, "Hope can be divorced from faith, but it is an empty hope." That is where we part company. George does not speak for me on that. I believe my hopes can be robust in the absence of a belief in God, if I can move beyond the skepticism that has been such a part of who I am for so long.

The poet Emily Dickinson was sent home from Mount Holyoke College in the middle of the nineteenth century, branded by strict Christian school officials as a "No-Hoper."

Dickinson had regularly rejected organized religion.

The event is captured in *A Quiet Passion*, a film chronicling the life of the controversial New England poet. "[Dickinson] didn't doubt [God's] existence so much as question his intentions," wrote A. O. Scott in a *New York Times* review of the movie.

Yet one famous Dickinson poem is strangely hopeful.

> Hope is the thing with feathers
> That perches in the soul,
> And sings the tune without the words,
> And never stops at all,
>
> And sweetest in the gale is heard;
> And sore must be the storm
> That could abash the little bird
> That kept so many warm.

Emily Dickinson was a godless woman, a rarity in Christian society of the mid-nineteenth century. She was unabashed in her dislike for religion but clearly believed in the power of hope. Hope could survive the storms of life. Dickinson was a secular thinker.

The suggestion that hope must be tied to a belief in God brings me back to square one. For me, that just seems exclusionary. "To some extent it is exclusionary," George said. "It is." The man is unapologetic about his perspective. I suppose if George did not hold strong convictions, he would be in the wrong line of work.

I wanted to find common ground with these two Jesuits, but I could not bring myself to embrace their belief system. Months later, when I remembered David likening hope to self-regenerative human immune cells, a light went on in my head. I emailed him, suggesting the comparison supports my theory that hope is organic and flowers on its own with no need for any particular belief system.

David responded the next day. "It does feel like a gift," he wrote. "That is, something that is beyond our own power or control to create. In that sense, it would seem to be 'beyond' natural, or to use the classic philosophical category, metaphysical. As this territory is beyond what science can measure and test, this is why I use mystery as the appropriate expression."

I relate to that. If hope really is inside us from birth and a natural human instinct, it does not require religion to activate it. Hope will be there for us to call on in our darkest moments. Finding hope within ourselves is the challenge. For many, there is no instant route to hope, no words from a text that will get us there. Hope is the continuum of a life story in progress. We must engage in a process, really a dialectic, and trust that it will gradually lead us where we want to go.

However rugged the detours, soft and slippery the ground beneath my feet, I do want to get there. If the search for hope takes me down a long road, I must stay on the move. I must accept that my destination is unknown and perhaps far away. I understand that and find joy in my own journey. My bags remain packed.

CHAPTER 12

Dr. Sadiq and the Magic Stem Cells

A few days after leaving the ancient city of Rome, I was back in Manhattan, waiting to walk through the door of the Tisch MS Research Center. The place was founded by Dr. Sadiq in 2006, and for me, he held the keys to the kingdom. I had called the office as soon as I could when we returned. A receptionist told me they were expecting my call, and I was immediately given an appointment.

I saw it as a good sign that the staff had expected my call. I knew I would be cutting in line if I became Sadiq's patient; by all accounts, there was a long waiting list. I was not counting on anything. I had heard stories of patients cooling their heels for close to one year before being seen by this man. Yet here I was, having been offered an appointment within one day. That told me Sadiq was serious when he invited me to see him. Why, I was not sure.

I was vibrating with anticipation and determined to engineer a seismic shift in my struggle to find health. After I had abandoned conventional therapies, my strategy for waging war on MS had been to sit in a rudderless boat and wait for a current to carry me somewhere. I was weary of doing nothing and accomplishing the same.

The center houses both his clinical practice and the research lab he directs. Together, these operations occupy tens of thousands of square feet in a large building on Fifty-Seventh Street, on the far west side of the city. With clinic and lab under one roof, this place offers its own version of one-stop shopping.

I am not inclined to take much at face value. I have been a journalist too long for that. Had Dr. Sadiq really wanted me to show up at his office, or was he humoring me as the conference ended? I had no reason to doubt him, but when things seem too good to be true, they often are.

According to the center's website, Dr. Sadiq has the largest MS practice in the world. The place is like an indoor stadium, noisy and packed with patients and staff. Locked doors separate the enormous research area from the more modest space dedicated to the clinical practice. It is not clear whether the lab rats are being locked in or the patients, who rarely get to see the research facilities, are being locked out.

The clinical area looks as if it houses an insurance agency, though there is an energy that one would not feel in a boilerplate business. Everyone walks quickly, as if preparing to race for the cure. I sat in the waiting area looking around. Patients chatted and appeared at ease. Neurologists and nurses actually smiled.

In short order, a receptionist ushered me into Dr. Sadiq's private office, where he was waiting. He walked around his desk and pulled up a chair facing me. Dr. Sadiq seemed relaxed, and the room was as sunny as he was. The door was closed, shutting out the noise from the corridors.

"I didn't think you would come," Sadiq said with a smile, as I sat in a modern chair and stretched out my legs. "Why not?" I asked, taken aback slightly. He shrugged and said, "Because I know how you feel about neurologists." I looked him in the eye, a little nonplussed, though he was correct. I did remember once telling him that no neurologist had ever done anything for me, to which he had replied, "Then you have the wrong neurologist."

I explained that I had walked away from conventional care months ago because it was not getting me anywhere; traditional treatments had become wasted exercise, like running in place. He said nothing, waiting for me to go on.

The usual drug protocols had yielded little, maybe close to nothing, I told him, and for years, my expectation level had been hovering around zero. I added that I was now ready for any sensible plan that might move me forward. I was hinting at cell therapy, but he did not immediately take the bait.

Sadiq's phone rang, startling me. He walked over to a table and answered, proceeding to engage in an animated conversation in a language I did not recognize. When he sat down again, I asked what he was speaking. "Punjabi," he said.

How many languages do you speak? I asked. "Six," he answered nonchalantly. Sadiq explained he was of Indian descent but hailed from Kenya. "Everyone over there speaks something different. You just learn them." I smiled as I thought about my own ignorance of foreign languages.

As Dr. Sadiq settled back into his chair, I had the distinct feeling he was glad to see me. He patiently waited for me to continue. Finally, I said, I am very interested in cell therapy. I think we both said at the Vatican that cell therapy is the future of medicine. Then I shut up, wondering if I was coming on too strong. I was ready to leave the past behind and hobble into the future. I did not know much about Sadiq's involvement with stem cell therapy or whether I would be a candidate for that kind of treatment.

Sadiq casually mentioned that he was awaiting a decision by the Food and Drug Administration on his application for a phase-one clinical trial using stem cells to treat multiple sclerosis. Those were the words I was hoping to hear. When he saw my eager face, however, he told me that he had been waiting a long time for a response. I know the FDA is a hard sell, so I took that as a warning to slow down.

That, of course, ought to be the MS-patient mantra. Do

not get your hopes up. Count on nothing. The landscape seemed so bleak. Thomas Carlyle, the nineteenth-century Scottish historian, had labeled economics the "dismal science." I thought the phrase would apply more appropriately to neurology. After all, if the numbers do not add up, economists can alter their methodology. Flexibility is the key to their success. Try altering the central nervous system to meet expectations.

But Sadiq was optimistic—his constant condition, as I would learn in the months and years ahead. He was upbeat and positive, a happy warrior. As we continued to talk about his work and my experience with MS, I felt for the first time in forty years that I was with a neurologist who did not see me as just faulty wiring in a body deadened to sensation.

By now, we had been talking for more than an hour. Dr. Sadiq made it clear he was open to trying to help me but quietly insisted on going forward in a professional manner. "I cannot work with you unless you agree to become my patient," he told me. "We'll need to do a full neurological workup and an MRI. And there is the spinal tap." Sadiq paused. I remembered surviving one of those procedures decades ago as part of my original diagnostic workup. The stab in the back was a procedure I had not forgotten. Nor had I forgotten the terrible headache that followed.

While I was revisiting memories of that spinal tap, Sadiq continued. "Let's identify the problems first," he said. I know

what the problem is, I said in my head. I am a used car on legs.
"Commit to me for one year," Dr. Sadiq went on, "and if you
are not satisfied, we can shake hands and say we are friends.
And you can move on."

That was an offer I could not refuse.

In the coming months, I underwent many hours of tests,
some of them rigorous, a few scary, even to a veteran patient
like me. One of the tests was a two-hour MRI meant to check
out my brain and brain stem. I have survived my share of
MRIs, but have you ever been trapped deep in a thundering
machine and required to remain absolutely still for 120 minutes? I have a survival scheme inspired by a movie where a
character devised a strategy for enduring a long sentence in a
third-world prison. I close my eyes, and in my head I go to the
beach in the company of beautiful women. What happens on
that beach stays on the beach.

Then there was the dreaded spinal tap, the long needle
pushed deep into my back. Forty years after my first tap, the
needles are much thinner, the numbing agent more effective,
and the procedure surprisingly quick. It was not as bad as I
remembered. I lay with my head down for about thirty minutes, then got bored and went home.

The next test was anything but boring. It was a relatively
new procedure called evoked potentials, which sounded benign enough until I got to Columbia Presbyterian Hospital.
The test did not feel benign. I entered an old building at Co-

lumbia and went into a small laboratory. As wires and electrodes were attached in multiple places from head to toe, a technician smiled and said, "Don't worry. You will be okay." Right. Now I was worried.

An electric current surged through parts of my body, measuring conductivity. When we got around to testing my legs, the voltage lifted them off the table. The muscles tightened; my legs shook violently. I thought I was being electrocuted.

On a summer evening, Sadiq administered an extensive neurological exam. The workup was thorough, taking a full two hours and lasting past dusk. Two hours with a doctor. Who has done that? This was a much more low-key affair than the other tests. No fancy equipment required, just Sadiq's watchful eye.

He had me move my arms and legs, toes and fingers, in every imaginable way; told me to walk on toes and heels, with and without the cane, testing strength and stability. He even asked me to make strange sounds, as if I were an opera singer warming up. Sadiq later explained that he wanted to determine if the disease affected my speech. Then he evaluated my proprioception, the ability to sense where one's body is in space.

"Now, walk toward me," he instructed at one point. "Hold your arms out straight. Close your eyes." He is going to trip me, I thought. "Keep your eyes shut." He took my hands and walked me around the examination room. "Good," he exclaimed. "You know where your feet are. Not everyone with MS does." Dr. Sadiq smiled and told me to sit down. The exam was over.

Sadiq and I were now alone in the cavernous office. The others had left long ago. I glanced out the window. The summer sun was setting. I looked at Sadiq and asked, Do you ever go home? "Every so often," he replied without looking up. He put the chart on the examination table. "Usually I work six or seven days a week. We have a mission here. This is my life's work."

Without missing a beat, he asked, "Do you believe in God?" That threw me. No doctor I'd ever been treated by had gone near that subject. I fell silent for a moment. "I am more drawn to nonfiction than fiction," I finally replied. "No, not really," I reiterated. Sadiq was recording everything on my chart. Why do you ask?

"I need to know this," he explained. "I treat a lot of Orthodox Jews who have strong views and different beliefs. Sometimes it helps to know." This felt different from any other workup I had experienced. I stifled the urge to ask Sadiq if he himself was a believer. I figured that time would come.

I was aware that Dr. Sadiq is a Muslim; how religious, I did not know. He has an easy way about him. He laughs a lot. So do I. Who cares which direction he faces when he prays? I liked the man.

I was sitting at the end of the examination table, legs

crossed. The good doctor stood next to me. The room was really cold. Medical facilities always are too damn cold for me. I was glad to be wearing a thick sweatshirt. Sadiq was in short sleeves.

"Are you always cold?" Sadiq asked. Yup. "That is the MS," he told me. No kidding, I thought. Sadiq asked me what my biggest MS complaints were. I froze for what seemed to be a lifetime of deep thought. I felt suddenly sad as I tried to answer from deep within the secret cave in my head.

Images of loneliness and frustration flashed across my mind. In airports, I told him, I have to use wheelchairs because my legs no longer can carry me to distant gates. The skycaps who are supposed to wheel me to my destination often seem to operate on slow-motion automatic pilot. Sometimes that means leaving me arbitrarily parked at an odd angle, some distance from my travel companions. Often my back is turned to them, and I am unable to see them, ending up excluded from their conversations.

I feel like an inanimate object, a solitary figure. I wait on the concourse, horribly self-conscious in my aloneness. I am a child again, unable to take care of myself, hoping someone in my party will notice my absence and come get me.

Sometimes what is more painful than being ignored this way is being praised. I have no use for anyone who, usually out of discomfort with disease, blows smoke by announcing that I inspire. Please. In 2016, *The New York Times* Opinion pages carried an essay titled "I Don't Want to Be 'Inspiring,'" by John Altmann, who has cerebral palsy and makes a powerful point. He described sitting in an audience with a friend when he was in high school and being embarrassed by the speaker.

"At the end of the assembly, my friend and I were singled out by the speaker, who said something that people with disabilities hear often—that because I got around on crutches and she with a scooter, we were 'inspiring.' In that moment my personal characteristics, the people I love, the interests I pursue and the beliefs I hold became moot, and the fact that I have cerebral palsy and use crutches to walk became the entirety of who John Altmann is and what he is about."

How odd that a compliment can feel so wrong. Many cannot see beyond our disability, and we become our disease. Altmann goes on to say: "I want a world that is so accessible, where technology and medicine become so advanced, that all disabled people get the chance to opt out of their disability. I want a world where the social relations I forge with those who are able-bodied are not predicated on my disability."

That is a fond, if futile, hope in a culture that celebrates beauty and physical perfection. For those who are disabled or live with chronic illnesses or both, we hope for one outcome: we want to be normal. Please, God, let me be normal. The world does not see us as normal, however, and sadly that is rarely how we view ourselves.

In 2006, in Chronically Upbeat, my online column for *AARP the Magazine,* I wrote about the longing to be like everyone else: "Almost all who have lived with a serious chronic condition for an extended period know the unsettling sense of being marginalized by the chronically healthy around us.

"We are all too familiar with our own limitations, keenly aware of what others can do, as we watch from our seats in the bleachers. I will be a spectator until my last breath is drawn. Gradually and grudgingly we grow used to our second-class status because there is no way around it. These observations originate in my own head. They are not on the lips of others.

"We are not normal by any standard measure, even to ourselves," I wrote. "So many of us live in our heads, sometimes the only safe refuge we know. We are driven there by others, by employers and dates and even casual friends who can say the wrong things, even while trying to do right. And we retreat to our secret place, the unseen hangout where we can be ourselves without feeling we belong in the local freak show."

I did not even mention this to Sadiq, who has many patients far worse off than I. That is my private head game. I know I am fortunate that I am still on my feet. I cannot lose sight of that. Yet there is no pecking order to loss. We deal with our own realities and would be fools to constantly measure our emotional pain against that of others. I just stay silent.

I am put off by those who complain, as if they had been promised a better deal. I try not to beat my breast or take out my frustrations on others. This is my life. I own it. I take pride in handling my issues with grace and dignity. Sometimes how often I express my grievances is all I can control. The sick learn how to juggle, to pick and choose strategies and swallow most of the pain. I am not going to burden family and friends with my unhappiness. Yet sometimes I know deep down that I am a burden.

I uncrossed my legs and told Sadiq about the time years ago when Meredith and I took Gabe to Spokane to start his first job as a television reporter. We arrived with little time to spare and much to do. The clock was loudly ticking. This was a time of quiet emotion for all of us.

We had to move quickly to buy a car, find an apartment, choose furniture and bedding, stock up on kitchen supplies and life's odds and ends. All this had to be done in little more than forty-eight hours. We needed more functioning arms and legs. There was no time for my physical shortcomings. I was useless, perhaps even an extra weight at a time when we could not handle more baggage.

As Meredith and Gabe headed down miles of aisles shopping for his new life, I was left in the dust. My presence was forgotten. With every stop I was quickly done in and went quietly out the door. Waiting in the car with only an FM radio station to keep me company had become a way of life for me. Meredith and Gabe were only doing what they had to.

I get it, but I never get used to it. I can walk only short distances and even those with difficulty. The world is in a hurry, but I cannot be. I could not keep up with my family that day. With my damaged eyes I had watched my loving companions melt into a distant blur. My life is an impressionist painting, a tapestry of fading colors and vague shapes.

I also remember the night Meredith and I were having dinner with Gabe and Lily and a few of their friends from Northwestern at a favorite restaurant in Chicago. My temperamental bladder suggested I find a restroom. Our waitress had noticed my cane and told me that I could avoid the long, steep stairway by taking an elevator down and heading into an adjacent building.

The young woman led the way. Once we had descended, she unlocked a heavy door connecting the two spaces and said she would wait for me. I moved into the next building by myself, stumbling and glancing off the doorframe. I ignored the pain in my arm. Bumping into inanimate objects had become a ritual. Bruises were a constant part of my life.

When I got to the bathroom the waitress had pointed to, I discovered it was locked. I was annoyed and retraced my steps, only to find the door back into the restaurant locked too. I just stared at it in disbelief. I was now focused on controlling my bladder, one of the little life crises that go with multiple sclerosis.

The corridor was deserted. I knocked. Nothing. I banged on the door in desperation. I really did have to go. I was standing there stone-faced when the door finally swung open. The young waitress smiled and told me she was just checking to see if I was done. I was done, all right, sick of these situations and tired of hoping for better.

Sadiq was scribbling, taking everything down. This doctor in his starched white coat wanted to know my priorities. I knew he genuinely wanted to fix all that was wrong with me, but as I sat on the examination table, I found myself slipping back into a cynicism born of hurt. I worried that Sadiq might join every other doctor and fix precisely nothing.

What did I hope for that day? I did not know. The exact nature of this exercise in wish fulfillment was not clear. For all these tests and visits to the center, there still was no plan. Sadiq had told me about his application to the FDA for a stem cell trial but had not indicated whether I would be included. That had been months earlier. The subject seemed to have gone to sleep.

After the tests were done, Meredith joined us. We discussed the results and talked about where we would go from there. Cell therapy was the elephant in the room. The idea was not mentioned. Meredith liked Sadiq, but agreed with me afterward that he had been vague about what would happen next. Our shared radar had picked up no signs of movement. And just like that, hope was stalled.

CHAPTER 13

East Meets West

I was in a Manhattan bar, talking to a friend who is Protestant by birth. I raised the subject of hope, and he had little to say. Catholics and Jews seem to run the show in New York City. Protestants are just a spiritual oligarchy without power. I thought of one place where I had crossed paths with thoughtful Protestants. That was Harvard Medical School, an unlikely venue for give-and-take about God. A small group of prominent physicians regularly met with a local minister to discuss issues of religion. These gentlemen were in their eighties, and I took them seriously.

On a hot, humid summer day later that month, I was on a train headed for Boston. My destination was the medical school campus at Harvard University, famously located on Avenue Louis Pasteur.

This was familiar turf for me. I had traveled there any number of times when I served on the advisory council of the

Harvard NeuroDiscovery Center, which did expedited research on five neurodegenerative diseases, including multiple sclerosis.

As I arrived, I made the same observation I always do, noting how imposing the complex is. Five large white marble buildings are grouped in a U shape around a long grassy quadrangle. The individuals I had arranged to see were two physicians I had worked with when I was on the council.

Dr. Joseph Martin is a neurologist and former dean of the Harvard Faculty of Medicine. It was he who had created the Harvard NeuroDiscovery Center. Joe had an interesting religious background in the Mennonite faith, a historically strict Protestant sect.

Dr. Timothy Johnson is the former chief medical editor for ABC News and a retired member of the faculty at Harvard Medical School. Tim was raised in the Evangelical Covenant Church, an offshoot of the Lutheran Church. He attended the University of Chicago Divinity School for a while and graduated from the North Park Theological Seminary in Chicago. He was ordained in 1976. After two years in the ministry, Dr. Johnson enrolled in medical school and later received a degree in public health from Harvard.

Tim is a serious man, but his years of working with newspeople have imbued him with a slightly irreverent sense of humor. We occasionally met for coffee when he was in New York, trading ideas and bad jokes. Tim always has a smile on his face.

Joe and Tim are freethinkers—men I respect. I remembered them as men of faith. "Two old Protestants," as Tim put it in a conversation with me. They always had been able to merge the scientific and the spiritual in an apparently seamless fashion. As I would learn in our meeting that day, though, each had struggled with faith, and there were hints of uncertainty in their views.

I like uncertainty. It is a badge of an honest person. I was to meet Joe and Tim for an informal lunch in Joe's office on the third floor of Gordon Hall, the handsome Doric-columned building at the head of the medical school quadrangle. Gordon Hall is the essence of old Harvard, with high ceilings, cast-iron pillars and railings, and leaded-glass windows—the highest of which are decorated with geometric patterns. Framed photographs and historical text decorated the lower walls, documenting the history of the medical school.

· Joe's office was a cramped but comfortable space where we sat eating sandwiches and trading stories. Our get-together that day had the quality of a reunion, and we reminisced for a while before getting down to business. It was Tim who brought up the topic I had come to discuss. "I was raised in a very conservative environment, both theologically and socially," Tim said. "Part of that construct involved very specific teachings about hope. As a child, I really believed with my whole being and heart that I was in the hands of God and therefore had hope for everything, for my life and for the world in general."

Tim's wording suggested that his childhood vision had morphed into something different. "At this point in my life, I have a very different theological construct and a much more informed, realistic notion." When he paused, I leaned toward him, eager to pull the words from him. "I still retain the belief that there is a supreme being of some kind in charge," he said. His tone was soft and steady. "The hope is rifled with doubt, but it is still there. I doubt as much as I hope, but when my back is up against the wall, hope wins out."

In his book, *Finding God in the Questions*, Tim wrote about his spiritual struggles and discomfort with his own Christian identity. In an online interview around the time of publication he said, "I don't often label myself as a Christian. So more and more I say I am a 'follower of Jesus.' You don't have to subscribe to all the intellectual, creedal developments of the Christian church and certainly don't have to support so many of its terrible choices over the years."

Many tend to fall back on the ideas we grew up with, but during Tim's time at the University of Chicago Divinity School, he was confronted with a theology and approaches to the Bible that were very different from what he believed as he grew up, which led him to a crisis of faith.

That was the start of a spiritual evolution that he still wrestles with today. His honesty about the need to give up some of his long-held beliefs is no mean feat. Living with doubt and uncertainty can be emotionally risky. People of faith must feel vulnerable when they turn their backs on what they once held dear.

Tim wrote about the pain of that in his foreword to Granger E. Westberg's book *Good Grief,* which is about finding hope and healing after serious loss. Tim had met Westberg, a chaplain and Lutheran minister at the Chicago Divinity School, when he was in the midst of his crisis of faith.

"I was struggling with my faith journey as it was being vigorously challenged by the intense intellectual atmosphere," Tim wrote. "My struggle was both physically and spiritually upsetting. I was grieving the loss of my simple childhood faith." I can see that once faith has escaped, it has to be very hard to get the genie back in the bottle.

Tim wrote that his recovery of faith was protracted and slow. He attributed part of his healing to Westberg, whose wisdom and words helped him, as Tim put it, "understand what I could believe—and to live with what I couldn't understand."

After hearing Tim speak of his struggles with faith, Joe, who had been listening quietly, jumped in. Joe is a gentleman, an endangered species in our culture. His white hair and upright bearing lend him a dignity that he wears, even in semi-retirement, every day. Yet Joe has the down-to-earth demeanor one might expect of a farm boy from Alberta, Canada. His roots are there. The cover photo of his memoir, *Alfalfa to Ivy,* makes that plain. The snapshot captures him standing in a field, wearing jeans and a checked shirt, holding what looks to be a baseball cap. The doctor and professor had gone home.

Joe's faith journey was long. His beliefs have changed radically. Perhaps this is because Joe's Mennonite faith has traditionally made fewer adaptations to modern life than many Protestant sects do, though many mainstream Mennonites are indistinguishable from the general population. Old Order Mennonites ride in horses and buggies and speak Pennsylvania Dutch, a language similar to German.

I asked Joe if his ideas about church doctrine had changed since his childhood. "For sure," he responded immediately. "I think it has been a transition over many years. You cannot be a scientist without discarding much of the doctrine religions have thrown at us."

Joe is a true scientist whose allegiance to empirical truth is stronger than that to any religious doctrine. But he made it clear that he still has faith. "I am not an atheist who believes the creation of the world just happened," Joe said. However, the beliefs he holds today are very different from the blind faith of his youth.

Joe questions the very foundation of his old belief system. "I can no longer conceive of the anthropological image of a figure that is supreme. I think we have to move closer to something that represents intellectual honesty rather than hypothesizing things that can never be proven."

This was not what I had anticipated on the train to Boston, and I wondered if Joe still believed hope had to be based in faith. "That is a very, very good question. I cannot say I can give a quick response to that." Joe paused and broke eye contact. Perhaps that was an answer. I knew I had to return to the question later.

I told Joe and Tim that I had asked Rabbi Kushner about his view of hope in the absence of faith. Kushner had rejected the necessity for playing the faith card in the search for hope. "I believe in hope detached from faith," Rabbi Kushner had told me. "When things are bleak, the best thing to do, rather than collapsing under our burdens, is to say that there is the potential for something good to come out of this that will make me stronger." That is a powerful view of hope. I noticed Tim nodding in agreement.

"I know people of no faith at all, sometimes with virulent feelings of atheism, who have very hopeful natures, even optimistic natures," Tim said. "More important than any religious feeling, there is a genetic biochemical kind of hope that we are born with to varying degrees." The notion of hope as existing in our DNA, "self-regenerative," as Reverend McCallum had put it, is reassuring.

I contacted Tim later to ask for clarification. "For some people, just as important as any religious feeling, there may be a genetic component, which is to say that our genetic makeup not only plays a major role in our physical health but also in our mental and emotional health. And for some people with strong religious belief, that can override the genetic determinant."

Joe and Tim made it clear during our conversation that they do not believe any individual or faith has a lock on spiritual truth. Their own faith had changed over time because they had kept their minds wide open, so they understood that faith has to be a very personal thing.

When I said goodbye to Joe and Tim that day, I no longer felt so alone with my doubts. The two had been clear enough about their own uncertainty that I felt they were singing my song. One question that was left unanswered was what I had posed to Joe Martin about the relationship between faith and hope. I emailed Joe a few weeks later to follow up.

"Faith for me is ambiguous," Joe wrote in response. "I do not have any sustaining hope that comes from a set of religious beliefs. I no longer find it helpful to believe that some form of intercessionary prayer or calling out for help will change the course of events." Joe went on. "I have been thinking about hope as a gift."

That word *gift* keeps coming up. If hope is a gift, is there anything we can do to encourage its presence in our lives, or does it just happen to us? A gift from where? I ask. From God, perhaps. Back to square one. I do not need to believe in a deity to be spiritual or to stake a claim to hope.

Joe Martin's final words during a telephone conversation caught my attention. "If I had a choice, in the sense of being born into a faith, Buddhism would be the place to be." That statement was a surprise from such a committed Christian as Joe.

I long have been curious about Buddhism. I thought about my Buddhist friends who are free, unencumbered by doctrine. I was not sure if they would say they believe in hope, but they do seem capable of a kind of calm in the face of suffering that does resemble hope.

I contacted Gopal Sukhu, an associate professor of Chinese at Queens College in New York. We have mutual friends. Gopal is a follower of Theravada Buddhism, or Doctrine of the Elders, which scholars generally believe contains the earliest surviving record of the Buddha's teaching.

Theravada has been the predominant religion of Southeast Asia for centuries and in recent years has begun to take root in the West. Today Theravada Buddhists number well over one hundred million worldwide. I figured Gopal would be a good person to answer my rudimentary questions about Buddhism.

The doorman in our Manhattan apartment building called to say Gopal was on his way upstairs. I had never invited a Buddhist over for coffee, and I half expected to see someone in sandals and with a shaved head. When I greeted Gopal at the elevator, I saw that he was wearing street clothes, not robes.

As we entered the apartment, Gopal stood still for a moment. He seemed transfixed by a large photo of a young novice Buddhist monk in Myanmar hanging in our entryway. The young man looked like a boy. His shaved head was smooth and bright. The man-child was wrapped in a saffron robe that covered him completely. He stared out from the wall with clear, welcoming eyes, as if allowing us to enter his world.

I felt I needed to explain to Gopal that the photo is simply an image Meredith and I find powerful. I am not a Buddhist and in fact I know very little about the practice. I was not even sure if Buddhists believe in a god. "No," Gopal told me. "We do not. The Buddha believed that religious ideas, and especially the god idea, have their origin in fear. The Buddha says, 'Gripped by fear, men go to the sacred mountain, sacred groves, sacred trees, and shrines.'" Amen. I liked this guy already.

In *Smile at Fear: Awakening the True Heart of Bravery*, Chögyam Trungpa, a Buddhist meditation master and scholar, wrote that the time has come to discard old myths. "We also have to give up the notion of a divine savior, which has nothing to do with what religion we belong to, but refers to the idea of someone or something who will save us without our having to go through any pain." No pain, no gain. "In fact, giving up that kind of false hope is the first step."

Gopal comes from the kind of religious background Trungpa was implicitly rejecting. Gopal's father, he told me, was Indo-Trinidadian, and his mother was an African American missionary. They had met in the late 1940s when she lived in Trinidad with her Christian missionary mother and Navy stepfather. That sounded like a Rodgers and Hammerstein musical to me.

Gopal's parents raised him Catholic. "I was baptized and

received Holy Communion. I was well on my way to Confirmation when my foster grandmother's sailor boyfriend arrived back from Hong Kong with books on Asian religions like Confucianism, Daoism, and Buddhism." And the hook went in.

For Gopal, Buddhism is all about exploration. "Buddhism is a religion of gnosis. The adventure in Buddhism is to see what you will find out. That is the opposite of the doctrinal approach of other religions. It is up to you to learn." That anti-doctrinal approach makes Buddhism different from any faith I know.

I asked Gopal about the concept of hope in Buddhism. He seemed dismissive of the hope game: "You can hope or not hope, and the result will be the same. The hoping does not bring it about." He did, however, acknowledge that hope can enable people to act in such a way as to help bring about the result they desire.

"The interesting thing is that hoping may give you strength. Some people need that," Gopal said. "From a Buddhist perspective, anything you need to do to get the strength to act, to move in the right direction, is good. There is flexibility. There is the belief that something will happen."

I wanted Gopal to explain how Buddhism helps people deal with a fear that, in other belief systems, can drive them to a belief in God. I do know a bit about that kind of fear. Awakening from a seven-hour cancer surgery with no idea what the results might be took me to my worst-case scenario.

If you cannot turn to God in such moments, I wanted to know, how do you find hope? "Being without hope is not the same as despair," Gopal answered. "Instead, it is, let's see what happens. That is the essence of gnosis."

The word *Buddha* means "awakened one," someone who has awakened from the sleep of ignorance and sees things as they truly are. Buddhism teaches the reality that sickness, old age, and death are the only certainties in life, the three eventualities a person can count on. Nothing more, nothing less. This seemed a rather grim approach to life, and after Gopal left I wondered why so many cheerful, happy people are so attracted to Buddhism.

I was learning to coexist with ambiguity, spending more time with questions than answers. I decided to reach out to one more Buddhist, Sharon Salzberg, who is a leading voice of Buddhism in America. Salzberg is the author of many books, including *Real Happiness* and *Lovingkindness*. In 1974, Sharon cofounded the Insight Meditation Society in Massachusetts. She has been leading meditation retreats around the world for more than three decades.

I met Sharon at her apartment just off Union Square in Manhattan, a neighborhood that attracts street vendors, protesters, chess players, chanting Krishna followers, and breakdancers doing their thing. I love passing through that carnival, and it is closer than California.

Sharon was friendly and ready to engage. I had told her in

an email that I had questions about both hope and faith. Sitting in her living room, I went straight to asking what faith meant to her. "Faith is defined as offering one's heart," Sharon said, "giving it over to something. But it has nothing to do with doctrine. It is faith in one's own inner capacity no matter what."

And hope? Sharon paused and smiled. "One of the things we pursue is an excruciatingly precise use of words, to the point of pain. So what does *hope* mean? In Buddhist teaching, when the word *hope* is used, it is not the way we use *hope* [in everyday life]." So how would a Buddhist define *hope*? The question seemed obvious. "It is a movement of the heart," she said. "Engaging, not sitting on the sidelines feeling marginalized. It's putting yourself in the center of possibility."

I believe I have tried to live my life that way, though I had never connected the task to Buddhism. I have embraced threatening conditions and held them close, recognizing that hideous possibilities are a part of life. Know illness and position yourself to fight. Participating in the stem cell clinical trial, whatever the terms of engagement, brought me face-to-face with a fact of my life. There is nowhere to run, no place to hide.

Sharon seemed to be saying that hope may not find us. We have to work to find hope. She believes there is an approach to hope that is different from what Rabbi Levy sees. Naomi believes hope can come to any individual open to it. Sharon also talked about the concept of attachment and made a distinction that seemed similar to the one Rev. David McCallum had made when he talked about not confusing hope with expectations.

"In the Buddhist sense, attachment means clinging or grasping," she said. "It suggests wanting to be in control, needing things. Attachments mean narrowing our playing field as if there is only one resolution." I believe what Sharon means is that fixing on a specific result is a bad strategy. Knowing there is a range of possible solutions and being able to accept whatever comes is a better mind-set for moving gracefully through life.

Mindfulness and meditation are tools that Buddhists use to let go of their attachments to specific results. Sharon thinks that mindfulness can also help us overcome worn-out thinking that limits our sense of possibility. "I look at hopelessness and its relation to mindfulness. We are so weighed down by old habits of mind. People tell us about ourselves. We internalize. We have a false sense of our limits. Sometimes it's manufactured, and mindfulness can reveal all of that to us."

Sharon recommends twenty minutes of meditation each day. "It's what one of my teachers called exercising the letting-go muscle," she told me.

Learning the power of acceptance is really what Buddhism is all about. And even though I know I am not very good at it, I understand how necessary that is for all of us, especially for people facing difficult life crises.

CHAPTER 14

The Great Bone Marrow Harvest

A few months after my thorough examination by Dr. Sadiq, I had another appointment with him. That day, as I climbed down from the examination table, Sadiq, unprompted, spoke the magic words: *stem cell therapy*. He told me he believed an answer to his application would be coming from the FDA in a week or so. I waited for him to say something else, but that's all I got.

I wondered if Sadiq was optimistic about the trial being approved. He was inscrutable, offering no hint of what he expected, though I thought I saw doubt in his eyes. For the first time since I had known him, Sadiq appeared weary. His entire life was built around finding the cause and cure for MS. It dawned on me how much was at stake not just for Sadiq's patients but for Sadiq himself.

"If I don't discover the cause of the disease, I will consider myself a failure," he had told me during one of our discussions in his private office. He meant it, I was certain. I had tried to point out that he gives so much to patients. Doesn't that count for anything? I asked. He just shook his head.

The following week, in mid-August, Sadiq got word that the trial had been approved. It had been three years since he had applied to the FDA. I happened to be at the MS center the day after news of the trial hit the wires. The air was electric. The office had exploded in excitement. Happy voices still echoed down the corridors of the clinic and throughout the research facilities. Everyone seemed thrilled. Phones rang out in celebration. Even the lab rats were smiling.

The news was a big deal. The press release the MS center sent out was picked up by newspapers around the world and was all over the Internet. "The Tisch MS Research Center of New York announced today that it has received Investigational New Drug (IND) approval from the Food and Drug Administration (FDA) to commence a Phase 1 trial using autologous neural stem cells in the treatment of multiple sclerosis (MS)."

Sadiq was widely quoted: "To my knowledge, this is the first FDA-approved stem cell trial in the United States to investigate direct injection of stem cells into the cerebrospinal fluid of MS patients, and represents an exciting advance in MS research and treatment." One medical newswire called the trial "a groundbreaking strategy . . . for the treatment of MS."

Sadiq had gotten what he wanted. I was happy for him,

but had no clue what it would mean for me. The man of the hour had a huge patient base, with lots of folks to choose from. I stayed silent, carrying around a lump in the pit of my stomach. I was in and out of the center that day and saw Sadiq briefly, but he didn't offer anything about whether I would be involved in the trial, and I did not ask.

One afternoon, Sadiq invited me in for a meeting in his private office. What he said blew me away. He told me I was at the head of the line. I would be the first MS patient in the world to be treated with mesenchymal stem cells (MSCs), infused directly into the spinal column. The stem cells would be harvested soon from the bone marrow in my chest.

This was huge. Processing the news was difficult. No matter how intrigued I had been about stem cell therapy since the Vatican conference, that tired old wheelchair was still parked in a dark corner of my mind. Suddenly my life felt different. It was as if I had crossed a finish line when I was only in the starting blocks.

I had a marathon to run, but was fooling myself into believing this would be a sprint. I was scanning the horizon, looking for the winner's circle. I never learn. I was ready to vault into my Triumph TR3 and speed away, leaving the wheelchair in the dust.

The trial would be an investigation, Sadiq explained, as I tried to bring my racing mind back to the moment. Phase-one trials are intended to assess the safety of a drug or device. But the treatment would be real. The trial would not be randomized, meaning there would be no placebos. All patients would be treated with the real thing.

A clinical trial is experimental, Sadiq cautioned, with outcomes unknown. But in my mind's eye, I could see only success. This procedure was new, and I was thinking big. Sadiq ran through a litany of disclaimers that go with an untested therapy. Volunteering to venture into the unknown is scary. But because the trial would be using autologous cells, meaning those from my own body, there would be minimal risk of rejection or other complications. People do not reject their own cells. There was no doubt, no fear, no hesitation in my head. I was ready to go.

"Are you certain?" Sadiq asked. Yes, I practically shouted.

Sadiq later explained why he thought I was a good candidate for the trial. "You present in an unusual way," he told me. "Most people have problems on both sides of their body. Only your right leg, arm, and hand are affected. That will make it easier to track change." I did not care why I had been selected. I was in.

That was what mattered. Sadiq's optimism was infectious. More than once, he had suggested that the stem cell therapy might allow me to put my cane away. He was not overpromising. He predicted nothing for certain. Sadiq just brings a positive energy to his patients, a hope that lifts them. When a doctor feels good about a patient's chances, why wouldn't a sick person feel at least a jolt of hope?

In fact, I was high on hope. Preparations for the trial were going full throttle, and I was acting as if I were oxygen deprived. My judgment had gone goofy. I was used to losing control of my body but not my hold on reality.

Hope had run amok. After years of adopting cold realism as I considered my life, I let my imagination fly. I was soaring. In my head, Meredith and I were walking the streets, climbing the hills of Rome. Ben and I were playing our second set in a tennis match without end.

I knew that letting my imagination go wild was a recipe for disappointment, but that didn't change the fact that my pent-up hope had built to the point of bursting. I was a pressure cooker waiting to go off.

On a Saturday in September, just weeks after Sadiq had gotten the FDA approval he needed, I went to the center for the bone marrow aspiration. The procedure was the first critical step in the process and would be the most invasive. Bone marrow, home to budding stem cells, would be harvested from my sternum, the breastbone. Meredith and Gabe and their cameras joined me for this hideous-sounding procedure.

I was overly concerned about the procedure. My legs quivered ever so slightly as I got out of the car. My pulse quickened when I stepped into the street. This is silly, I kept telling myself. But my characteristic calm, the equanimity, was cracking. I reminded myself that I had survived worse.

Walking through the doors to the MS center, I glanced back. The old CBS Broadcast Center was located directly across the street. I had spent years working in that former fly-infested dairy, and it had been an important part of my identity. Familiar turf as it was, now the place struck me as remarkably unfamiliar. For a moment, I was haunted by my past. Then I readied myself to step into the future. I felt like a page was turning.

Nervous energy merged with excitement as Meredith, Gabe, and I stepped into the elevator. The closer we got to our destination, the tighter the knot in my stomach. Part of me dreaded what was waiting upstairs. However, there was no thought of turning back.

No pain, no gain, I reminded myself. I had endured so many awful medical procedures for MS and colon cancer. Nothing under the sun should have unnerved me. When I was a young man, I allowed a medical resident to inject steroids under an eye, directly into the eye socket, in hopes of treating my failing optic nerve. I've had an angiogram that almost blew my head off. But here I was, quaking in my boots that an expert in his field would soon be mining for gold in my chest.

It was a Saturday, and the reception area that morning was quieter than usual. Dr. Sadiq sees patients on weekends, so there were people in the waiting area, and a small group of his staff was there to greet us as we got off the elevator. Gabe was lugging video equipment, ready to document the procedure for my *Journey Man* blog. Another camera crew joined us, this group videotaping the procedure for the MS center. The offices was being transformed into a movie set.

We headed into Sadiq's sunny offices. I had never minded going to that place for routine appointments, since his staff was just as bright and sunny as it was outside the windows. But there was nothing routine about this day. Soon a hematologist, a blood doctor, would arrive to screw a strange device into my breastbone. Poke yourself really hard in the chest and see how it feels. Then do it with something that I imagined to be similar to a corkscrew and stop wondering why my knees were knocking.

The objective was to capture the mesenchymal stem cells within the marrow. As Sadiq had explained, mesenchymal cells are a type of stem cell typically located in the bone marrow of the sternum. The hope was that when the harvested cells were later infused into my spinal fluid, they would travel to the lesions—the trouble spots in my brain and brain stem—where they would repair the affected neurons and protect my immune system from further attacks on the myelin sheaths.

Five months after the Vatican conference, I was about to embark on the journey I had heard so much about in Rome. I still could not stop the flow of fantasies, the notions of recovered function through this strange new process. I knew scientists around the world were using stem cells to create new organs in laboratories as well as to combat diseases. I wanted those cells. I wanted to run and to hike again. I wanted to regain my lost vision, even to drive a car again, something I had given up long ago.

As we waited for the hematologist, Meredith turned to a nurse, who was busy arranging instruments. "How painful will this be?" she asked. The young nurse paused and looked toward the ceiling. "Oh, it's not really painful," she told Meredith. "It will sort of feel like his chest is being crushed." I was so relieved.

Soon the hematologist, Dr. Gabriel Sara, arrived. He was a middle-aged man with an Eastern European accent. I did not ask him where he was from. Sadiq greeted him, thanking him for making a special trip on a weekend just to treat me. Dr. Sara seemed good-humored, smiling broadly when I introduced Gabe. He checked his supplies and busied himself, preparing to dig deep.

I removed my shirt and lay back on the table. Before he began, Dr. Sara calmly described each step of the procedure he was about to perform. He would numb me first, then numb me again before screwing a surgical instrument used in extracting the bone marrow into my breastbone.

As the device went into the bone, it would open a narrow passageway into the marrow. At that point, Dr. Sara would remove the top of the surgical instrument and put a syringe in place to aspirate the marrow. The whole procedure probably would take no more than fifteen minutes, he said.

Dr. Sara made the procedure sound routine, and I began to relax—at least until I saw the device he would be using. I had been expecting something hideous and was not disappointed. The thing really did look very similar to the corkscrew I had imagined, but with a long, straight needlelike pipe rather than a spiraling piece of metal extending from the end of it. God help me.

We were under way too quickly for me to dwell on the device. Dr. Sara placed a cloth over my face. It was like being hooded before my execution. He told me he wanted to shield the point of entry from coughs and sneezes. If I were claustrophobic, I would have lost it right then. The cloth did have a small hole for my nose so I could breathe.

Activity began with a familiar stinging pinch, lidocaine, a local anesthetic being injected into the skin at the site. The doctor then did it again, this time pushing deeper. "Do you feel any pain?" A little, I mumbled. Dr. Sara paused, probably wondering if I had bothered to answer. I decided to get a grip. He continued. "Sometimes it takes a few minutes."

When satisfied that I was numb, he began to screw the large corkscrew into my breastbone, as if opening a bottle of fine wine. I felt pressure but nothing more. As he kept screwing in the device, the pressure in my chest continued to build. This was going to be trouble, I was sure. But there are no pain receptors in the sternum, so it was not as bad as I'd imagined.

"Okay," the doc finally said. Okay, what? I asked. The aspiration? He paused. "Yes. The aspiration," came the dreaded reply. Say goodbye to my wife and kids, I thought. This was the piece of the process I had been warned about. The aspiration would be the big bang, the explosion heard 'round the world. The doctor was about to stop pushing in the plunger. Now he was going to pull it back, extracting a significant amount of blood containing vast quantities of bone marrow. From this eventually would come millions of stem cells, more than a lifetime supply.

I felt mild pressure and waited. The pressure mounted. Here we go, came my silent cry. My chest tightened. Meredith stared into my eyes through the small breathing hole in the mask over my face. What are you looking at? I hissed. Before she could say a word, the doctor looked up and said simply, "Okay." Okay what? I thought "The procedure is over," Dr. Sara told me. What? I want my money back, I thought. This was what I worried about for weeks? I asked softly. The smiles around the room made me feel silly. As usual, the anticipation was worse than the reality.

By my count, I had injected myself with various MS drugs close to a thousand times, with little more than sore arms and legs to show for it. Perhaps there was hope in the contents of Dr. Sara's syringe. As soon as I had that thought, I checked myself. Why would I allow myself to feel anything so positive and upbeat?

Charlie Brown was foolish for believing he would ever get to kick that football, when all of us kids knew Lucy would pull the ball away at the last second and poor old Charlie would swing his leg at air and land on his ass. Blind optimism is a ticket to nowhere, so I felt a deep need to protect myself, to harden my shell and continue to doubt. I did believe in Sadiq because I knew his credentials and trusted my instincts about him as a human being. But I could not bring myself to assume anything else. I just could not.

"You know you are a pioneer," Sadiq said to me one day when I was in his office not long after the aspiration. I knew he did not mean that I was a hero but simply that I was participating in a groundbreaking experiment, attempting to treat a disease that never has been controlled before. Yet Sadiq's words sent a powerful message. At least I was doing something positive. Meaningful. How liberating, I thought. How novel. It felt good to be on the front lines, to be part of the first wave going ashore. Fear of failure receded as excitement took over once again.

Most people do not know the daily grind of awakening in the dark and testing their legs to see if they will be in working order to allow one more day of life in an upright position. Now I was not just in the audience, waiting and watching. I was onstage, ready to write my own review.

There was nothing more for me to do at this juncture. While doctors and technicians completed the elaborate process of cultivating the stem cells that had been harvested, I had at least three long months to wait for the next step, the first of what would probably be several stem cell infusions.

I was curious about the part of the process that didn't

involve me, so I emailed Dr. Violaine Harris, who supervises the lab, to ask her what goes on behind those closed doors during the months of preparation for the infusion.

"Bone marrow cells are separated from red blood cells with a centrifuge," she replied. "The purified bone marrow cells are cultured in a petri dish and kept in an incubator. The cells are grown in a liquid supplemented with a nutrient-rich sample of the donor's blood."

Mesenchymal stem cells are large cells resembling brain cells, able to perform much of the work of the 210 cell types in the human body. MSCs stick to and grow on the bottom of the petri dish. In approximately two weeks they fill up the petri dish. MSCs are then expanded several times to obtain enough cells for cryopreservation. "Prior to the stem cell treatment, a portion of the MSCs is thawed and expanded again to 100 million blank cells," Harris wrote. "After about three months, these cells are infused into the spinal fluid of the patient, and the treatments are underway."

What we were embarking on sounded like a hunt for a miracle to me, though I do not believe in such happenings. I wondered if Sadiq did. By now, I knew Sadiq was a religious man. "I do not use the word *devout*," he told me one day. I was glad to hear it. That word felt like it had a bad connotation in this era of extremism. "But I do believe in God."

Sadiq was easy to talk to and not at all self-serious. "I will make you a bet," he suggested. "If you get better, you start believing in God. If you don't, I will become an atheist." Sadiq laughed, quickly adding, "I don't think I can do that." This is a man who faces Mecca, sometimes with the help of a compass, and prays as many as seven times each day.

What happens during those prayer sessions? I wanted to know. "I just communicate with God, who I believe is the creator of everything," he explained. "But I don't believe in dogmatic religion, and I certainly don't believe in those who are killing people," Sadiq declared, seeming to pick up speed. "They are barbarians and worse than or as bad as Nazis. I mean, those are just complete lunatics. I don't believe in that kind of religion at all." I had sort of figured that.

Sadiq and I were sitting in his private office, talking and eating tiny pieces of candy that kept getting stuck in my teeth. Of course I complained. "You have to rise above it, Richard," Sadiq told me. I assumed he meant to focus on more important things. "I am a Sufi Muslim," he went on. "We are mystics. My family is from India. This is common there."

Sufism is a mystical form of Islamic belief and practice. Sufi Muslims seek to find truth and divine love and knowledge through a personal experience of God. Sufi Muslims are said to focus on issues of human importance.

I asked the good doctor if he belonged to a mosque and regularly attended religious services. I was picturing a neighborhood house of worship in suburban New Jersey, where he lives. Sadiq paused. "I lead a service at a Christian church in

Manhattan, actually near here. I just quietly leave for a while on Friday afternoons. The staff here doesn't even know."

I asked him why he would lead a Muslim prayer in a Christian church. Until recently, he said, the prayer group had met in the basement of a local hospital. But then their numbers had gotten out of hand and they needed to find a new space. One day a patient who worked at the nearby church had offered to introduce Sadiq to officials whom he could speak to about the possibility of holding Muslim services there. "We'll just come to pray, and we'll be in and out in two hours if you give the church to us every Friday," he had told the officials. They said yes.

I asked Sadiq if I could go with him and attend Friday prayers. I knew nothing about Muslim rituals. I had seen footage of massive prayer meetings, the faithful bowing to the earth in unison. I wanted to experience this in a more intimate service. "I will take you sometime," Sadiq answered.

CHAPTER 15

The Power of Human Decency

I was deep into my search for opinions about hope. This was not a scientific study, only a mission that might mean something to me. Already I knew there was no single answer to any question on my mind. Perhaps this was only a self-indulgent exercise. But my different conversations were compelling and instructive. I was seeking perspective, not expecting wisdom. I needed only a friendly voice on the phone. My problems were piling on. I felt very alone. I wanted to touch and be touched.

I was determined to seek out individuals who had stared down trauma. January 29, 2006, was the day Bob Woodruff and his wife, Lee, saw their world explode. Bob was the newly installed anchor of ABC's *World News Tonight*, the successor to Peter Jennings, who had died of lung cancer the previous year. Bob's first assignment took him and his cameraman to Iraq to cover the war. A few days after their arrival, they were out shooting a story just north of Baghdad when a roadside bomb ripped into their armored vehicle.

Both newsmen were grievously wounded. Woodruff sustained catastrophic injuries to his head, face, and neck. He had suffered a traumatic brain injury. There was so little hope for his survival that his producers in New York began planning his obituary.

Lee Woodruff, to whom he had been married since 1988, learned of the blast in an early-morning phone call from David Westin, the president of ABC News. As she recounted in their memoir, *In an Instant*, when Westin told her that Bob had been wounded, she asked him, "What do you mean *wounded*? . . . Is my husband alive?"

Yes, Westin told her, but he had taken shrapnel to the brain. "I tried to digest what that meant and couldn't comprehend it," Lee wrote. "He was alive; I'd start with that. The rest was gravy." The simple fact that Bob was alive was enough for Lee to reach out and touch hope. It was not much, but it was something.

Later in their conversation, Westin told her that when Woodruff regained consciousness, he, too, asked if he was alive. Hearing that her husband had awakened and even spoken was grounds for further hope, she felt. "So he spoke, I thought. He spoke. This is going to be okay," Lee wrote. "Bob would be okay. He was lucky and bright and hardworking and a good man. Things like this didn't happen to good people. I could feel hope in my heart, as clear and bright as the streak of a shooting star."

Bob Woodruff underwent surgery at a U.S. Air Force hospital in Iraq before being airlifted to a hospital at the U.S. Army base in Landstuhl, Germany. From there he was flown to the National Naval Medical Center in Bethesda, Maryland. Doctors kept him in a medically induced coma from which he did not emerge for five uncertain weeks.

I had crossed paths with Lee in 2008, when she interviewed me about my second book, *Strong at the Broken Places*, for ABC News. I decided to reach out to ask Lee if she and Bob would talk to me about the hope that sustained them during that trying time. I did not know Bob, nor could I anticipate how they would respond. Lee wasted no time getting back to me, letting me know they would be happy to talk. They were gracious and accommodating.

Lee invited me to come to their home in a suburb north of New York, straight across the county from the village where my family lived. Lee, an author and a freelance writer who did gigs on television, greeted me in their driveway, wearing jeans and a sweatshirt that read, "I Love Sundays."

It was a warm, sunny spring day, and we sat out back, looking at the view of the ocean, with Long Island visible in the distance. It was just the two of us, since Bob was on assignment for ABC. I asked Lee how she had managed to find hope while her husband was still unconscious.

A kind of denial seemed to come into play. "I didn't know a lot about brain injuries, and that saved me," Lee said. "I very early on understood that if I wanted to stay in the world of hope, I should not find out more about brain injury until he came out of his coma."

On the videotape in your head, I asked, were you seeing Bob recovered or not? "What a great question," she quickly replied. "On the videotape in my head, I think I needed to play the tape both ways so that I could begin to get used to it, however it was going to break."

Lee told me that she is a person of faith. She had leaned on that faith when she had a miscarriage and subsequent hysterectomy in 1995. Faith, she told me, had pulled her through that ordeal. But when she found out what had happened to Bob, she wondered if her faith would be strong enough to sustain her again, especially if the news was grim.

In an article she wrote for *Guideposts* magazine a year after the explosion, Lee described what her faith had meant to her during a time of such uncertainty. She wrote about how the prayers of friends and family and even strangers had sustained her ability to hope when her own faith sometimes wavered.

As a person of no faith, I asked Lee if she felt one has to be a believer to find hope. Do you think hope is organic, that it can grow, even if you are not someone of faith? I asked. Do you believe everyone has equal access to hope?

"I do, Richard. I really do," Lee said, becoming animated.

"Let's get back to your word, *optimistic*," Lee said, referring to a word I had used earlier in our conversation. "People who would register as more optimistic are probably able to tap into their hope more easily," Lee said. "I think some people are probably more predisposed to being hopeful than others."

That could be a mixed blessing. Optimism can lead to expectations, sometimes unrealistic. If a person in need is seduced into believing that if you hope hard enough, the desired end will come to pass, then the expectation game can be dangerous. Lee, however, thinks the alternative is worse—that not having hope leads to despair.

"The absence of hope is a much scarier place to be and I believe a less positive place from which to heal and move forward," Lee told me. "I think despair is crippling. It is somebody frozen and incapable of movement. But moving forward is the only choice we have if we want to grapple with our new realities."

That did not mean Lee had not known moments when she felt frightened and unsure. By the time her husband was airlifted to the States, the doctors thought he would survive. But in the weeks Lee was with him at the Naval Hospital, while he was still in a coma, his prognosis was unknown, his future uncertain. A military physician described his condition in guarded terms: "The question is, what kind of individual will we have at the end of this period?" For Lee, the uncertainty about just who would emerge from the long sleep was agonizing.

"The doctors said he might be violent, that sometimes people recovering from brain trauma hit their loved ones. They said he probably wouldn't ever be able to do his job again. Please, God, I prayed. I just want my husband back."

Lee had been clinging to the fantasy of wounds healing and full restoration. Revising that to "I just want my husband back" meant that she was trying to adjust expectations. Lee still had hope, even if it was dimmer. When Bob had not emerged from his coma after nearly five weeks, that hope, too, began to fade. The doctors told Lee that Bob would have to be moved to an acute-care facility.

Just as the dark clouds began to take over, the sun broke through. Lee went to Bob's hospital room one morning and was shocked to find him sitting up in bed. "Bob had awakened on his own, as I was at my very lowest moment, when I think I was pretty much out of hope. 'Sweetie,' he said, 'where have you been?'"

As Lee wrote in *Guideposts*, "This was so much more than I'd wanted and prayed for, that I couldn't really believe it. My husband was back and he was calling me." Bob was back, but he had a long road ahead. Recovering from a traumatic brain injury is a marathon, not a sprint.

Half of Bob's skull was gone, with his brain protected only by skin, so later he had to have surgery to replace his missing skull with an acrylic plate. Memory issues and cognitive deficits became the new normal, at least for a time. Doctors told the Woodruffs they would just have to wait to see how fully he would recover.

Some weeks after my conversation with Lee, when Bob returned, he told me the story of what he had experienced during the long months of convalescence and rehab. Bob described the raw emotion that frequently overtook him. "I just cried and I couldn't stop. There are all sorts of brain issues that trigger things that are not natural. Everything from anger and snapping and that kind of thing," Bob said evenly. "They did not tell me that a traumatic brain injury is permanent." The old normal was gone.

"When I woke up, I couldn't remember the names of a couple of my kids," Bob said. "I couldn't say *paper clip*, I didn't know how to say *coffee* or especially *decaf*. I couldn't even order something from Starbucks when I finally got out of the hospital."

I told Bob I did not speak Starbucks either. He laughed. Bob's sense of humor seemed to have remained intact. His friends tell me he is an incurable practical joker. I can relate to Bob's need to laugh. A sense of humor is a valuable coping mechanism. "Laughter is a form of internal jogging," Norman Cousins, the legendary magazine editor, wrote of his battle with illness. "It moves your internal organs around. It enhances respiration. It is an igniter of great expectations."

I think of all that Meredith and I have endured together over the years. My medical meshuggaas has veered out of control from time to time. When MS and cancer were foisted on me, it was a struggle to laugh. I was too freaked out. Meredith knew how to handle that. My good wife informed me she had purchased a cute black dress. "Just in case," she added, putting on a grim face. "You will love it, except you won't be around." Relax, dear, I responded. I'm not dead yet. Laughter releases internal pressure.

There is a wonderful video of Bob Woodruff lying in bed with his young kids around him. The children are teaching Bob to pull words from his faltering brain and relearn how to pronounce them. They made it a game. Bob was clearly comfortable allowing his children to take the lead. Whether or not he truly needed their assistance, the video presented a moving picture of a family coming together to support one another.

Bob described the long path he had traveled to recover practical brain function. "I had to go through all these tests where they give me little note cards with a picture of a hammer to see if I could say the word *hammer*," Bob said, "which I couldn't. I couldn't remember the different kinds of fruit. I didn't know what that yellow car thing was. It was a taxi."

One month after that conversation, I sent Bob an email, asking him to detail the cognitive deficits that remain. "Remembering words," he replied. "Mild aphasia (an impairment of language, affecting the comprehension of speech and the ability to read or write). No small obstacle for a journalist."

He continued, "I can make my points with different words

if I forget certain ones. Names are more difficult because there are no synonyms." I asked if he thought he could anchor again. "I suppose I could," he wrote. "But not exactly the same way I was." Woodruff has residual deficits from his injuries, but he has made an extraordinary recovery, having moved far beyond the point where doctors warned that his progress might end. He was back on the air within thirteen months of the explosion, though not in the anchor chair.

Woodruff knew he was fortunate to have had the finest possible medical care for the injury he incurred in Iraq. He and Lee decided they would do what they could to make certain that men and women in the military also received the help they needed. In 2007, they formed the Bob Woodruff Foundation, which raises money and provides grants to programs assisting veterans and their families. Their mission statement reads, "We will pursue ways to provide service members and their families access to the same quality of support through their recovery that Bob Woodruff and his family received."

By the end of 2016, the Woodruff's nine-year-old foundation had invested forty-two million dollars in various programs to help wounded veterans pay for rehabilitation costs and get educational and employment assistance after leaving the service. The Woodruffs have found a way to bring meaning to the trauma they survived. Their commitment to helping is now built into their lives.

Helping others with the same or similar issues becomes a

means to elevate our lives and escape the dark hole that can swallow us. I have spoken all over the country about my battles with disease. That mission has helped me, probably more than anyone stuck in my audiences. Reaching out is rewarding.

Bob recounted being in the military hospital and seeing people suffering even worse injuries than his and thinking, "Why is this? It is not fair. If there is something we can do to help some of them, why can't we? So, yes, I found good in the bad."

This idea of finding good in the bad reminded me of what neurologist Oliver Sacks brought to his patients. Sacks was a physician who knew how to look past the conventional medical assessment of the deficits from which his patients suffered. Unlike most doctors, he understood it was possible for a patient's problems to "play a paradoxical role, by bringing out latent powers, developments, evolutions, forms of life, that might never be seen, or even be imaginable, in their absence," as he wrote in *An Anthropologist on Mars*.

When he was dying from liver cancer, Sacks discovered his ability to find renewal and strength, "new forms of life," as he wrote during his ordeal too. In an op-ed for *The New York Times* in early 2015, Dr. Sacks wrote about his impending death.

"I feel intensely alive, and I want and hope in the time that remains to deepen my friendships, to say farewell to those I love, to write more, to travel if I have the strength, to achieve new levels of understanding and insight." A powerful coda to an anthem of hope.

B ob Woodruff was blindsided by a bomb, causing a traumatic injury to his brain. Tom Brokaw did not see cancer coming until his world was upended by a rare condition and his grip on life imperiled. Tom is a highly regarded journalist— he anchored *NBC Nightly News* for almost two decades, until 2004—who happens to be a good guy too, often its own rare condition. I like Tom and have always found him accessible and open. I was working with Dan Rather, the anchor of *CBS Evening News*, when I first crossed paths with Brokaw in the lobby of the Savery Hotel in Des Moines during the 1984 Iowa caucuses. The bitter Great Plains cold radiated up through the soles of our shoes to our ankles.

In Iowa, all of us were onto the same story. The economy in the state and across the country was faltering. Unemployment was high and interest rates were through the roofs of farmhouses across the state. Everyone covering the presidential campaign that year was attending farm auctions because farmers throughout Iowa were losing their livelihoods. Thirty years later, Tom was in danger of losing his life.

In February 2014, Brokaw disclosed that he has multiple myeloma, a rare cancer affecting blood and bones. The announcement of his illness was jarring. Multiple myeloma had taken the lives of former vice presidential candidate Geraldine

Ferraro and ABC News anchor Frank Reynolds, my advocate during my earliest years in television news.

I later ran into Brokaw at *60 Minutes* regular Bob Simon's funeral. Tom was characteristically friendly when I saw him. He looked thin, even gaunt, wearing a suit that seemed too big for him. I asked about his health. "I am in remission," Tom told me cheerfully, then asked about my health. I told him I was okay. Neither of us went into any detail. This was neither the time nor place.

In early 2016, I sent Tom an email to ask if he would talk to me about hope. "Of course," came the quick email reply. "Given my own experience, I, too, have been thinking a good deal more about the subject." Not surprising. The topic had to be front and center in his mind.

Brokaw's public reaction to his condition had been typically understated. He chose not to indulge in melodrama, instead putting his focus on the good fortune he has enjoyed through the years. "In the seasons of life I have had more than my share of summers," he wrote on the first page of his new memoir, *A Lucky Life Interrupted*.

When we spoke a few weeks later, we talked about his new struggle. You have enjoyed more than seven decades of good health, I said to the NBC veteran. Getting hit by the cancer truck must have been shocking, so beyond any expectation that it must have been like being the victim of a hit-and-run driver.

"It was, and you have known me long enough and well

enough to know that I really have been a lucky guy. Everything has broken my way. When I have bumped up against stuff, it's been resolved. So I was conditioned to believe [chronic illness] is not going to happen to me."

I believe all of us rationalize and try to put a brave face on situations, I said. We have our hiding places until we have to face facts. "I think that's true," Tom responded. "I think in the life you and I had before we were diagnosed, the glass always was half full. I thought this would be an extension of that." Of course a glass half full can empty before you know it.

Brokaw told me about going to the Mayo Clinic in Minnesota to have some tests because he was showing disturbing symptoms. When the studies were finished, a doctor called him in. The man was blunt. "I know I can be candid with you because you are a journalist. And we have to make some moves fast," the doctor said to him before presenting a diagnosis.

When I asked Tom how he had responded, he thought for a minute before saying, "It was kind of an out-of-body experience. My first thought was, Okay. I have cancer. Then they [the doctors] said, 'You know, people have died from this.' I processed that and asked, how long do I have? They said, five years technically, but we think you are in good shape, and we might be able to extend it."

The way Brokaw told me about that moment, it was as if he had stepped out of his body and was covering his illness as a news story for NBC. He was dispassionate as he described the scene with his doctor, talking facts, not feelings.

181

Tom is a smart guy. He had to know exactly what he was up against. I wondered how well he processed reality when he got the news. "Intellectually, I understood I had cancer," he said. "But emotionally, I thought I had gotten through so many things in the past." Tom cited a helicopter crash, a near-fatal boating accident, tours in Beirut and Iraq and Afghanistan. "I assumed I'd make it . . . I probably thought I was immune."

There appeared to be no dents in the Brokaw armor. Tom sounded disarmingly positive. He had the self-confidence of being the captain of his own ship—someone who is always in control, the person who has the power to choose what to cover, to do things his own way. It looked as if he had control even now. I marveled at his calm. What did he know that I didn't? I wondered.

You seem to have taken on your illness as a journalist, I said to him. It sounds as if you are in a little bit of denial. "I think so," Brokaw agreed. Whether he thought that was a positive or a negative, I could not tell. Tom had answered with no hesitation, no discernible emotion.

I believe denial often is an instinctive reaction to bad news. Denial can be a good thing if it gives one ammunition to stay in the struggle. For fighters, denial is a powerful weapon. When we deny the inevitability of probable outcomes, that denial can partner with hope. Denial also can become a liability if it defies common sense. Tom learned that the hard way.

Tom's ability to keep a lid on his dread about his illness is even more impressive given that his red cape fell apart the day after he returned to his Montana ranch from the Mayo Clinic. "Here I was, just diagnosed with an invasion of my bones. I felt pretty good and drove one hundred and fifty miles to go fishing." That is difficult for a New Yorker like myself to wrap his mind around. "By the next morning, I was in fetal position on a cabin porch in so much pain I could barely move. Two days later, they were medevacing me back to Minnesota." Wishful thinking had overtaken reason.

By the time I spoke to Tom, he was already a couple of years into his ordeal, and I wondered if in retrospect he thought denial had served him well. "Most people who have been diagnosed with cancer just take it to DEFCON 1 immediately," Tom said. He paused. "Cancer means I am going to die." After a deep breath, he went on. "I am an optimist. I am not going to die. They said it was treatable. I'm going to try to stay in that corner of the diagnosis." The power of the mind must be harnessed when fighting a deadly disease.

Tom does know that denial has its limits. There has been no turning away from some of the complications cancer has caused, including painful fractures in his spine that had to be repaired. "This was a signal to me like pages of a book or a description from a physician on how the cancer had invaded my body in a more profound way than I had realized." Reality had set in.

For both Tom and me, our families—strong wives and loving children—have been a crucial piece of our survival strategy. Tom's oldest daughter, Jennifer, is an emergency room physician and has served as his point person in the wilds of modern medicine. Tom's wife, Meredith, to whom he's been married for fifty-five years, is his rock. "I think you know my Meredith enough to know she is a lot like yours. She is very stoic. When I delivered the bad news, she just stared at me. She was very analytical."

After our conversation, I wrote an email to Tom with one follow-up question. If you had asked me what I hope for, I said, I probably would say as long a life as is possible and to get to have and know my grandchildren. What would you say? Tom answered, "My hope is much the same. I would only add that I hope for a long productive life, more time with my grandchildren, and not to be an undue burden on my family."

Pretty standard, I guess, but Brokaw continued: "I have learned that my position in life and my experience with cancer and the culture surrounding it has made me a resource for so many others—and I am grateful I can be helpful."

Bingo. Becoming an advocate, an activist or, in my case, a guinea pig for others soothes the spirit. Hope comes in many shapes and sizes. Helping others is a high calling. I asked Tom if he felt his illness had given him a new sense of his life's mission. "I didn't anticipate that I would become a kind of poster boy for MM," he wrote back. But he was in a perfect position to fill that role by virtue of being a household name and using it for the good of others.

"I'm in regular contact with a Navy admiral, a Dallas Cowboys coach, a friend whose brother is struggling with MM, an assortment of strangers who stop me on the street to compare experiences. I don't offer medical advice but we do exchange treatment protocols, symptoms, surprises."

Dealing with illness and injury had pushed both Woodruff and Brokaw to new levels of self-awareness and insight. Both were different after what they endured. They probably were better human beings for their ordeals. Each thought it important to reach beyond his struggle and think in larger terms. Both were hoping to find meaning in all they had endured. I believe the ability to find meaning in personal battles is a form of hope, that selflessness eases the pain.

Some months later, I was hearing through the CBS News grapevine that my pal Allen Pizzey actually had pulled the plug on his time at the network, as he had told me at the Vatican he planned to do. I did not believe him then. Everyone in the business talks big about getting out from time to time, but in the end keeps their boots on and tied.

I knew that if Allen was leaving the network, his departure probably had something to do with the trouble he had been having with his eyes, which we had talked about in Rome. A few years earlier, he had gone to a doctor to have his eyes checked for what seemed to be a minor problem. The next thing he knew, his doctor was telling him to sit down.

"I like to be completely honest with my patients," the doctor had said. He then told Allen his diagnosis, that he was going blind and made the diagnosis of retinitis pigmentosa. Bam. I asked Allen if the news knocked him off his feet. "Not really," he answered.

Pizzey is a guy who made a living catching grenades in his teeth. He was unflappable. "I just went home and sat down in a chair. I looked around. I knew I needed to make a mental map of where everything was." Pizzey's survival instincts were automatic.

Now, after thirty-six years and assignments in about one hundred countries, Pizzey really was retiring. Who'd a thunk it? Pizzey's reporting had taken him to the epicenter of news in some of the world's most dangerous spots. He had covered the fall of the Berlin Wall and armed hostilities in Bosnia, Rwanda, and Kosovo.

Allen had been in the townships of South Africa in the age of apartheid, done tours in Iraq and Afghanistan, covered battles in Beirut. It has been said that journalism is the first rough draft of history. For millions, Pizzey's drafts had made sense of a violent, complex world. Now he decided it was time to choose calm waters over the turbulent seas he had been navigating for so long.

As he planned, Pizzey waited until his contract was up. I was trying to handle my situation with dignity and class.

Allen did just that. He sent his CBS bosses a letter announcing his intention to leave the network. "I've been elated, exhausted, terrified out of my wits," his letter read, "laughed, cried, reveled in adrenaline highs and suffered the lows of malaria and stomach bugs, been cold and dirty, coddled in luxury, logged hundreds of thousands of air miles. I've met villains and near saints, seen people do the most horrific, and heroic things imaginable, been awed by the kindness of strangers."

All in a life's work.

When I got back in touch with Allen, he told me that he knew it was time to retire because the damage retinitis pigmentosa had done to his vision had gotten steadily more severe. "I don't drive at night anymore. I don't like to be in crowds either, because I don't see people coming in from the side anymore. I bump into people. It's awful. I don't see down unless I am looking down. I walk into tables and trip over dogs and small children. It is annoying and embarrassing."

Forget embarrassing. Severely compromised vision would be dangerous to any person in Allen's line of work. "I used to go to war zones," he wrote to me in an email. "I know what you have to do. I've been in enough of them. Spatial awareness is really important. I'm either going to get myself hurt or killed or somebody else hurt or killed."

I wondered how Allen felt about having to give up the work he loves, which has been so central to his identity. "It pisses me off," he said when we connected by phone. I have been through the same thing, so I get it. I spent half my life battling illness and had to leave the news business decades before I felt ready.

Pizzey took a deep breath before adding, "I get angry at myself." So do I. Admitting to an illness can feel like a sign of weakness. Guys do not do well with that. But Pizzey also surprised me with an expression of hope, or at least a feeling that bore a resemblance to it. "If you are going to give up on something and say this has got me beat, you might as well end it. I am not going to commit suicide," Allen said, laughing before adding, "Yet."

His determination to hang in there may have had something to do with the fact that although the doctor in Rome had given him an extremely dire prognosis, an ophthalmologist he had seen in London for a second opinion had questioned that prognosis. That doctor told Allen that although he would have to learn to live with RP, he would die of natural causes before completely losing his sight. I, for one, have learned the art of being grateful to nobody in particular for small favors.

I asked Allen about his emotional reaction to the good news. I expected a description of whiplash. "Emotional reaction? Not very emotional at all, more a feeling—maybe even expression of 'Whooof. Okay. That's a relief.'" I should not have been surprised. Pizzey probably survived his life covering a cruel world because of his ability to suspend emotion. He had done that in response to both the bad news and the good news that followed.

Living with RP has meant that he's had to accept a lot of unwelcome change. Allen and I both know that many people have far worse problems than we do. Allen told me about a friend and colleague who had pancreatic cancer and was given a few months to live. "He said he was going to carry on as close to normal as possible. He was not going to sink into despair and drag people down. If he can do that, what I have pales in comparison."

Folks in the news business can be a cynical lot, well defended against the inhumanity and natural horrors we cover. How do our well-oiled defense mechanisms function when it is our own wounds we watch and weigh? I was struck by Allen's expression of humanity.

The determination to go on is an affirmation of hope. "A hero is an ordinary individual who finds strength to persevere and endure in spite of overwhelming obstacles," according to Christopher Reeve. Allen and I are no heroes, but I, for one, feel better about myself when I can find that kind of determination in myself. That strength only adds to my resolve to keep going. That gives me hope. My resolve had been cracking. Allen was helping me rediscover my grit.

Allen told me he planned to remain in Rome, which has been his home base for many years. His longtime partner, Dee, the mother of their grown son, Alexander, stays by his side. He takes daily walks along dirt roads and paths through woods and fields near his house, often spotting the occasional *cinghiale* (wild boar) or fox. Allen also plans to spend time at his house on a lake in Canada. The stakes for Allen are high, and he has chosen to live his life one day at a time, enjoying the things that have always given him pleasure. A sense of normalcy can breed hope.

Six months after our last conversation, I contacted Allen for an update on his condition. "I've developed a retinal edema, which is characteristic of retinitis pigmentosa," he told me. "I'm on a three-month course of drops to reduce it. If it doesn't work, they try an injection and then surgery. It's not getting any worse, so I'm hopeful."

I asked Allen if his life had changed. "I've curtailed some activities, but my life isn't a mess and I'm getting used to bumping into and tripping over stuff." And then this: "No sense bitching."

It felt good to talk to Allen. I identified with much of his positive attitude. Like me, Allen gets a lot of strength from his family. As with me, Allen had a father who taught him toughness. "My dad had no time for whining or giving up," he said. "I guess self-pity was never an option." I just smiled when I heard that.

CHAPTER 16

Stem Cell Infusion

This was a day I had been waiting for my entire adult life without knowing it even could exist. The morning dawned bright and clear. I was headed for Dr. Sadiq's office, where I was going to receive my first stem cell infusion. My rendezvous with the long needle was about to begin, and it might bring me a new life.

The infusion had been scheduled to occur three months after the bone marrow aspiration, which had taken place just weeks following the FDA's approval of the experimental procedure in August 2013. But before the timeline was certain, there was another hurdle to be jumped. Approval by the Tisch MS Research Center's Institutional Review Board (IRB) also had to be won.

The FDA acts on behalf of the public to determine when experimental procedures are allowed to be performed on humans. IRBs serve the same purpose on behalf of the institutions where these procedures are performed. Historically, IRBs exist to prevent unethical medical procedures such as the gruesome experiments conducted by Nazi physicians during World War II. The IRB's mandate is to protect the rights and welfare of anyone participating in medical research projects. An additional priority, left unstated, is to protect the institutions from potential lawsuits. IRBs are known to be cautious and conservative.

Even in the United States, there have been inhumane research projects performed, such as the Tuskegee Study of Untreated Syphilis in the Negro Male. In that study, 399 poor black sharecroppers who had contracted syphilis were tracked for forty years, from 1932 to 1972. Researchers wanted to see the natural progression of untreated syphilis.

When the study began, there was no treatment for syphilis. But by 1947, penicillin, an effective treatment, had been discovered. Yet the unknowing patients in the study were not offered the treatment so that the study could continue unencumbered. It was a national disgrace, and leaders of research institutions are trying to prevent anything like that from happening again.

One day Sadiq called me to say, "Richard, can you come in for a few minutes?" Invitations to chat with Sadiq in his private office were not unusual, so I was not alarmed. But the news he delivered was a shock. Sadiq had decided I could not be in the clinical trial. My stomach muscles tightened hard as he explained the problem.

My two bouts of colon cancer had disqualified me. Although specialists at Memorial Sloan Kettering Cancer Center had evaluated my case and cleared me to be included, I had been disqualified because of the possibility of comorbidity—the presence of two or more diseases that exist simultaneously and usually are independent of each other—which is a concern with any trial.

If I were in this clinical trial for MS and suddenly died of cancer, everything would have to grind to a full stop for an investigation, even if cancer had nothing to do with the trial. That would take time, and with trials, time is money. Sadiq had told me the total price tag for the phase-one trial was $1.5 million. Additional trial phases were expected to cost multiples of that. In the end, Dr. Sadiq and his colleagues were not going to take chances. I was toast.

As Sadiq explained the situation, I saw the bright future I had imagined disappear into dark clouds. I put on my usual game face. I got it. Just winning FDA approval can break the bank. Each phase of a clinical trial is hugely expensive. I had learned at the Harvard NeuroDiscovery Center that upward of a billion dollars can change hands before a drug or device wins FDA approval. There is no room for unforced errors.

Sadiq's news was hard to hear and absorb, but his demeanor was reassuring. He made this development sound like no big deal. He was a no-drama doc who would have sounded casual if my pants were on fire, though in this case, the smoldering was north of my neck.

Sadiq suggested an alternative. "I will treat you, and you will have everything those patients in the actual trial receive, but you will not be part of the official experiment." He paused. "Do you care if this is how we will do it?" I said nothing. But I did care. I wanted to be on the front lines of the battle, part of the first wave going ashore. Participating as an add-on took away that fantasy. I really wanted to do something for future generations. Perhaps my children, or their children, will someday be at risk. Beyond self-interest, lending a hand to those who follow is a coping mechanism. The desire to make a difference for future generations makes the pain of the present more bearable. That is a version of hope.

I had been appearing on television with Sadiq and in articles to publicize the trial. The publicity was intended to raise funds needed to keep the research going. It felt weird appearing as one of the public faces of a trial in which I was not actually participating.

Patients in the office had seen me on television with Sadiq and wished me well. I had written posts about the trial on my *Journey Man* blog, along with posting videos of some of the procedures leading to the actual stem cell infusion. What was I supposed to say when people approached me to talk about it? A more serious concern was that I might be putting Sadiq and possibly even the trial at risk by continuing to receive treatment even though I was no longer part of the study. That would have been unconscionable. After I returned home, I called an old friend for advice. Bradie Metheny has written extensively about National Institutes of Health and medical research issues. I explained the situation and asked if this kind of arrangement is common. He said he would look into it.

Bradie has sources at NIH. When he spoke to NIH officials, they assured him such actions were routine. "It has been going on forever," he reported back. "The reason is that doctors want to give patients the best they have." I decided to put aside my reservations, let go of my ego, and take yes for an answer. I just kept my mouth shut.

The Tisch IRB came through and approved the stem cell trial. Setting up the first infusion and performing last-minute checks in the lab would take a few days. I felt like an astronaut waiting to go into space. What difference would a few more days make when I had been waiting more than forty years to ride this rocket?

Less than a week after word came from the IRB, I was within hours of receiving my first stem cell infusion. I had been living with an incurable, debilitating disease for so long, and finally here I was. The journey had been arduous. Months of antibiotics and probiotics, gamma globulin, and other assorted drugs brought me to this moment. There was the never-ending blood work. For months I had been stockpiling blood in the lab at the Tisch center, preparing for the day that never seemed to come. Every time I went to see Dr. Sadiq, one of the nurses would tackle me and draw blood. I figured if I even walked through the Tisch center's neighborhood, a nurse would stalk me and stick a needle in to steal more of my blood.

"Blood serum is a rich source of growth factors," Violaine Harris, the lab supervisor, had explained. My blood was needed to feed the stem cells and act as fertilizer, she said, which would help them to grow and multiply. Now, if all had gone well in the test tubes over the past months, these cells would be coming out fresh and healthy from Dr. Harris's lab, ready to return to their natural home: my body.

I do not believe anything in life is meant to be, but somehow I had found myself in the best place for me at the right time. Pieces of an unlikely puzzle were coming together, and I was ready. I needed to believe in something, to see light over yonder. I pinned my tattered hopes to this shot in the haze.

A blustery wind coming off the Hudson River greeted my arrival at Sadiq's office. Meredith was at my side. There is a time for doubt and a time for hope. I felt the temptation of high expectations, and though I knew I should bat it away, I gave in. Even in the privacy of my mind I did not admit to the wave of hope I was feeling. Not in words, anyway. But a reassuring feeling kept bubbling up, and I did not resist.

Nothing special took place when we arrived. There was no ceremony to mark the occasion, not even someone to greet us at the door. Actually, no one paid much attention to us. For everyone else, it was just another day at Tisch. As soon as we were escorted into the treatment area, business got under way fast. Nurses appeared, schedules in hand.

I was surprised to learn that cognitive tests would be administered first, to establish a baseline for measuring possible changes in cognition from the stem cell infusion. Good, I thought, maybe that meant I could hope for the return of some of the pieces of my mind that seemed to have gone missing.

Compromised cognitive skills are common with MS. Over many months, I had become aware of my own cognitive deficits. Names and dates had been replaced by black holes between my ears. I had been trying to ignore this, but I knew the empty spaces were there. Brain slippage is scary, even when nobody else seems to notice.

I was led into a small office. Two clinical research assistants sat behind a desk with a number of strange-looking items on top, including a pegboard. The young women went through a description of the three tests I was about to undergo—all part of the multiple sclerosis functional composite test. Hadn't I seen this movie before? Concerns about cognition were not new, though they used to be easy to ignore. These tests promised to be as bothersome as the problem.

First, I was to take a math test. Math was never my strong suit, and it had not occurred to me that I would have to pass a math test to get a stem cell infusion. In high school, I was lucky to get a C in any math course. I smiled at the women behind the desk and reminded myself that life is not fair.

One of the assistants pushed a button to play the recorded directions for taking the test. Talking machines make me nervous. The device rattled off the instructions and offered to repeat the whole thing. That sounded like a good idea, and I listened to another run-through.

A series of numbers were read out at the rate of one every three seconds. I was to add the first two numbers I heard and say the result out loud. Every time the recording said another number, I was to add it to the last one I had heard on the recording.

One of the researchers elaborated when she saw the blank look on my face. "The machine will say nine, then one. You will say ten. The machine will say three. You will say four because three plus one, which is the last number the machine said, equals four. Right?"

I nodded and the test began. For a brief moment I thought I was doing okay, but the pace picked up, and soon I was flying down the mountain on greased skis. Fifteen minutes after arriving at the center, I felt numb. Couldn't we just do the freaking infusion? I silently asked.

The nine-hole pegboard was next. This provides a measure of upper-extremity (arm and hand) function. I sat there putting pegs in holes as fast as I could. Finally, there was a twenty-five-foot walk to test EDSS. That stands for "expanded disability status scale," a fancy term for seeing how long it takes to walk twenty-five feet. It's always part of the testing neurologists perform on MS patients, I guess because speed of walking is a factor that is easily measured and quantified.

I did not do well on any of these tests, and I did not care. I only wished to be reacquainted with my missing stem cells. Apparently my mediocre performance did not disqualify me from getting the infusion. A nurse came to escort me to yet another office, where I would have a cursory physical exam.

This quick once-over reminded me of a company physical that anyone who is breathing can pass. A doctor I had never met took my vital signs, casually asking if I had done the math test. Oh, yes, I answered wearily. He laughed. "I took it once to see what it was like. Totally incomprehensible." That was a relief.

After the physical, the doctor walked me to the treatment room where the actual infusion would take place. Meredith was there, waiting for me. The room already was busy, with men and women in blue scrubs walking in and out, looking at watches, carrying trays of instruments, fiddling with equipment whose purpose was unknown to me.

Because events would unfold quickly once the cells were brought over from the lab, everyone was feeling the pressure to make sure all the advance preparations had been made and everything would be ready to go. An expectant air hung over the space.

I felt as if I was the only person who was not tense, but when Sadiq came in, he was his usual relaxed self, smiling and joking with Meredith and me. Sadiq was a calming presence, but he, too, was busy. He tended to his preparations for a few minutes, then left the treatment room for a while. He came back and left again in short order. I assumed he was seeing other patients. He excused himself to check with Dr. Harris a few times. It was as if the stem cells were young children, and he was worried about their well-being.

As Meredith and I sat in the treatment room, we watched the men and women in scrubs bustling about. It was interesting to be surrounded by individuals so intent on what they were doing while we had nothing to do but stare into space. Eventually everyone finished their tasks, and one by one the medical staff left. Meredith and I were finally alone. Meredith grabbed her camera and began to interview me for my blog.

The primary objective of the blog was to connect patients living with MS or other chronic conditions. There is a longing among the sick to have a sense of community for support. We have heard enough from doctors and want to hear directly from individuals living with illnesses and enduring treatments. We want to compare notes and read about how other people cope. We just want to feel connected to one another.

Whatever I accomplished with Dr. Sadiq would be worth sharing with other patients. I knew that. He understood. I had never read any first-person accounts of stem cell treatments or the procedures leading up to them. I was sure this would be of interest to readers of my blog.

I had already posted the video Meredith and Gabe had shot of the bone marrow aspiration, and it had received an enthusiastic response and many thousands of views when it found its way to YouTube. I thought it would be valuable to record the infusion itself. Very few people know anything about how these infusions are done, and this was an opportunity to demystify the entire process. I also figured the video would provide a valuable record if I ever chose to write about the experience.

Meredith asked me how I felt. That was a softball question, of course, but it caught me off guard. I paused. "This is the day I get my first stem cell infusion. I have waited for this for a long time." I was surprisingly emotional, which left me unable to say anything more than that.

"But what are you thinking," Meredith asked, again catching me by surprise. She leaned in. "I don't know," I answered. I was not exactly eloquent. We have had much better conversations in our kitchen, but at this moment, I was overwhelmed.

"You don't seem to hold out hope," Meredith continued, baiting me for the camera. "*Hope* is a very difficult concept for me," I said. "It always has been. Experience had taught that the expectation game is dangerous. Disappointment always is something I try to avoid. I take things as they come," I added.

"You have to start somewhere," Meredith said softly. "Exactly right," I answered. I realized I was not ready for this conversation. I did throw out another thought. "I'll tell you, it's a step I wish I could have taken twenty or thirty years ago."

"Well, at least you have the opportunity to do it now." Meredith was right about that too.

Dr. Sadiq walked back into the room at that moment, and

I was off the hook. The introspection was abruptly over. Dr. Sadiq kept looking at his watch, all business. "When Violaine leaves the lab with the cells, we have only a certain amount of time to put them in you," he told me. "We want the cells to be alive." Sadiq had told us that already. His calm from a few minutes before had slipped away. Now he was wearing pressure on his bright blue sleeve.

"We want more than seventy-five percent viability," he said, meaning three-quarters of the stem cells had to be alive and kicking. Less than that meant he would not do the procedure at all. Sadiq was hoping for a higher number, 90 percent or so. The truth is, he explained, they had no idea what the optimum number of living cells should be. There is guesswork involved in first-time experiments.

This was a completely new procedure, and everything about it was an unknown, including of course, the results. All Dr. Sadiq knew for sure was that he was conducting an exciting experiment that might pay off. We were in this together. I felt relevant after all.

Sadiq was thoughtful as we waited for the arrival of the cells. "This is a little like buying a lottery ticket," he said. I agreed the stem cell infusion was a gamble but hardly seemed as trivial as that. Sadiq kept working as he spoke, looking over his instruments to make sure everything was in order. He examined vials of this and test tubes of that, checking paperwork and rechecking his watch.

"If you really care about the patients, you are moved by their desperation," he continued, almost as if he was talking to himself. Sadiq was letting down his guard in a way I had not seen before. "When there is not an obvious solution, you want to push the limits." The guy made it clear he was suspending expectations. "We get so much disappointment in research. We go down so many paths that don't lead anywhere. I want to drive forward, but I do not expect to succeed."

Excuse me? I did not take that statement at face value. I knew how much he cared and was keenly aware of the weeks and months, even years, that had delivered him to this moment. By nature, Sadiq is an optimist. He seemed to be playing the same mental game I play with myself, downplaying his hopes to shield both himself and his patients from disappointment. If he was not radiating his usual upbeat attitude, it had to be because he was weighed down by a hunger not to disappoint his patients. Self-doubt in a physician is refreshing. The moment was humanizing.

Still, his words as he ruminated certainly were making me tense. I wanted his steady hand on the needle as it entered my spinal column.

"I have no second thoughts about this. I have checked everything out. All the safety tests are negative, for cancer and everything else." He was covering his bases one last time. These assurances were another version of informed consent, though without the patient's signature. I already had signed my life away.

If the doctor was looking for a reaction, he did not find it. I sat stone-faced. We had covered this ground already. I just wanted to move forward. Sadiq seemed satisfied and continued with his checklist. He smiled impishly and reiterated a point he had made months ago.

"Now, you are a tall guy, and there are certain disadvantages to being tall."

"Not that I know of," I muttered, looking at the shorter man who would be wielding the long needle. "When we travel in economy class, I have a better time than you do," the doctor shot back.

Meredith started laughing, as did I. "And when we do a spinal tap," Sadiq went on, "you are more likely to get a headache than I am." I knew from experience that spinal headaches are killers. Meredith interrupted Sadiq.

"So when Richard gets home tonight, he should stay off his feet?" she asked, staring sternly at me. "Yes," Sadiq answered. "He should be lying down as much as possible." Great, I thought. "Do you hear that, Richard?" Meredith asked. "Are you promising that?"

I was not going to take that lying down. "I did not hear myself promise anything," I answered. Sadiq seemed to think that was funny. Meredith did not crack a smile. Sadiq's humor had made her laugh. Mine did not. Even as Sadiq kept chuckling, he made it clear he wanted me to play it safe. "If you get a headache, then don't call me," he said. "Okay," I shot back. "We have a deal."

"A spinal headache is worse than anything you've had," Sadiq warned me, "worse even than the leprosy you have right now." He laughed. Sadiq was referring to a mystifying skin condition that had started a few months earlier. Neither he nor anyone else could figure it out, never mind treat the pain. The itching and burning were out of control, driving me crazy. But at this moment, I thought we needed to break the tension, so I laughed too.

Meredith seemed to have decided she was not going to be distracted from the matters at hand. Aiming her camera at Sadiq, she put him on the spot. "Is there any evidence that this will actually help?" Silence. "No," came Sadiq's terse reply. A longer silence followed.

Once again, I considered how much Sadiq was risking. Years of hard labor, an entire body of research, and his reputation as a scientist were on the line. For him, the pressure would extend beyond this initial phase-one trial. Assuming the trial was extended, Sadiq had told me, the next phase would cost approximately three million dollars. Depending on the scope of what the FDA ended up approving for a phase-three trial, the cost for that would be even greater. It could be as little as twenty million dollars or as much as several multiples of that. The fund-raising would be intense.

"But you should ask a follow-up question," Sadiq said finally. The doctor looked up at Meredith, who kept the camera on him. "What question?" she asked.

"How many people have done this before?" he said. "And the answer is nobody in the world has received the kind of cells we are giving Richard." Man. Sadiq had a flair for the dramatic. His statement was sobering and at the same time exciting. This would be my shot. I was not about to turn back.

Meredith looked at me. "You are a pioneer," she said. "Or a guinea pig," I shot back. Silence. Enough talk, I thought. Let's get on with it. "The dog barks," a Persian proverb goes, "but the caravan moves on." The clock was ticking. Sadiq again left the room to check in with Dr. Harris.

The lab was just a few hundred feet from the room where we were sitting. Medical laboratories are strange, secretive places. I had never known what goes on in those mysterious places, where technicians walk around in white coats and wear surgical masks, passing through locked doors into rooms that are either freezing cold or unbearably hot. However, I had been allowed into the lab to get a view of the processes before a stem cell procedure. Violaine had showed me around, explaining that to determine how many cells were alive and well, she would take a small sample of them and place them on a slide under the microscope. She then would add a blue dye that permeated the cell membranes.

"If cells are alive, they will actively pump out the dye and appear white under the microscope. The dead ones appear blue," she'd said. By counting how many white and how many blue, she could estimate the percentage of cells that were still alive.

If the magic number had been reached, the plan was for her to grab the cells and sprint to my spine. And it really would be a sprint because the timing was so critical. The cells had to make their way from the lab into my spinal column in less than thirty minutes.

After his latest conversation with Violaine, Sadiq decided it was time to get me ready for the infusion. This meant inserting a catheter into my lower back. The needle carrying the stem cells would be inserted into that catheter, and the cells would travel into my spinal canal.

Dr. Sadiq had me sit at the edge of the examination table, still in my street clothes. My shirt was pulled up and taped into place so my back was exposed. The room was cold and the solution rubbed on my back considerably colder. I had to be germ-free and freezing at the same time.

I leaned forward into a pillow held by a nurse and arched my back. I needed to hold that position but was surprisingly comfortable. The prospect of getting stabbed in the back probably should have been unnerving, but I was calm. Before starting the infusion, Sadiq numbed my lower back with lidocaine. The injection felt like a bee sting. "Did you feel a pinch?" he asked. I said nothing, only nodded my head. He numbed it again just to be sure. Then he inserted the catheter.

I felt unsettling electrical sensations but no pain as he

worked. "That is the last sensation you should feel," Sadiq told me. Great. We were just waiting for the special delivery of stem cells. Everyone in the room sat quietly. I felt remarkably relaxed. Why wasn't I nervous, I wondered, or even excited? Now that the infusion was imminent, I felt nothing, which was disappointing. This moment had been so long coming. I felt detached, perhaps defensively. I just stared into space.

Actually I stared at the empty hallway. The door to our room had been left ajar, as if we were waiting for Elijah to appear for a cup of wine. Suddenly the doorway was framing not a prophet but Violaine Harris, who half-ran into the room with a smile on her face.

As Violaine skidded to a stop, I had a vision of her sliding into the wall and dropping the special transport vials. We would have been picking tiny parts of me off the floor, separating them from the shards of broken glass. Violaine shared the news that almost 95 percent of the stem cells were alive. We were ready to roll. Dr. Sadiq appeared relieved. "Let's do this," he said.

There had been so much preparation for this moment that the final scene was almost anticlimactic. "Now, Richard," Sadiq said softly, looking into the camera rather than at me, "I am injecting the stem cells back into you." The topical numbing agent he had injected earlier was still working, and I felt nothing. "I injected about three million cells," Sadiq told Meredith.

Dr. Sadiq repeated the infusions twice in rapid succession that afternoon. About nine and a half million stem cells found a new home in my spinal column. I knew in theory what the cells were supposed to do, and it was time for them to step up to the plate. We would not know how effective the process was for a while, if ever. There were no schedules, no timelines. Even under the best circumstances, I knew I was not likely to see changes for a long time.

"You did great, Richard. You are a very good patient," Sadiq told me when he had finished the final infusion. It sounded as if I was going to be given a treat and a pat on the head. But there was no candy. No brass band played. Simple satisfaction was the order of the day. The cells had a very high viability percentage, and the procedure had gone without a hitch.

Sadiq viewed the elaborate experiment as a success. He handed off a vial of something to Violaine, who had stayed to watch the process. Sadiq explained that she had to play around with the cells until it was time for my next infusion. "If you are still alive then," he said, adding, "just a joke."

All the joking hadn't obscured the reality that this was serious business. We were playing high-stakes stem cell poker, and the pressure was undeniable. My condition had been steadily deteriorating for a long time, and the manifestations were wearing me down every day. I longed for relief.

Yet I was not the only patient invested in the outcome of

the trial. That was apparent each time I hobbled into the Tisch center, leaning heavily on my cane. I regularly made my way past patients in wheelchairs or on scooters. Many of them had not taken a step in years. They had as much riding on this clinical trial as I did. I understood that I could not allow myself to lose sight of that sad fact. Many of them knew I was in the trial and had wished me well.

Today's main event was over, but after the infusion I had to spend close to three hours on my back, squeezed onto an uncomfortable, hard examination table taking the two IV antibiotics that were part of the protocol. The once-bustling room was now empty and silent. Meredith had departed as soon as the infusion was completed, but I could still feel her presence. A nurse occasionally stopped by to remind me to keep my head down.

Once the IV was finished, one of Sadiq's assistants gave me a tentative schedule for additional stem cell infusions. The FDA-approved protocol called for three infusions, spaced months apart. They would monitor me in the months ahead and perform some interim tests before giving me the second infusion. In the meantime, it was suggested that I should start taking iron pills, because I had given so much blood that I was now anemic.

When I finally left Sadiq's office, I was happy to be out in the fresh air. Maybe not all that fresh, since I was standing close to the West Side Highway. Everything around me looked good at that moment. I felt as if my new stem cells were giving me a new lease on life. It was not just a gift to me. My children and other patients might reap the benefits.

I owed a lot to Saud Sadiq. The rap on Sadiq has been that he overpromises patients. I do not see it that way. He is a glass-half-full guy. I think patients like and look for that. Signs of hope buoy us. Dr. Sadiq told me he would like to see me put away my cane, but he neither predicted nor promised that outcome. He merely believes it is possible. And that is what patients need to hear. The hopes of a doctor fertilize our gardens.

That optimism is not something I take for granted. The way many doctors and most patients see things is different; we are not coming from the same place. Doctors are protocol-driven, sometimes seeming to care as much about process as about people. Medical types can focus on charts and lose sight of the human body in the bed.

Patients need the human connection, which physicians often overlook or discount. That connection matters. Too many doctors have decided to focus only on the science of medicine, losing sight of the art of being a healer. They can be detached from its human consequences. Sadiq's patients are so loyal to him for a reason. We know how much of himself he gives to the people who have entrusted their lives to his care, and we know how much we matter to him.

Many years ago, the longtime chief of the New York City

chapter of the National MS Society told me that she hears patients complain about nearly every MS physician in the city. She said she never has heard a complaint about Sadiq from a patient. That tells you something.

I have crossed paths with physicians who have issues with how Sadiq conducts his research, and I know he is controversial. Fair enough. I do not have a dog in that fight. I do not even understand enough to be able to grasp what the controversy is about, so I cannot judge.

All I know is, this is a man whose devotion to his patients is total. Sadiq is committed to making our lives better. For us, that is what counts. Despite the few moments when Sadiq had allowed himself to express doubt, I knew he had high hopes for the stem cell treatment. The man's self-doubt did not reflect a crack in the science. My faith in what we were doing was whole.

The day had ended without news, but of course none had been expected. The race had only begun. Results would be tallied much later. My tolerance for ambiguity was serving me well. Uncertainty ruled the day. When I went home, I did keep my head down. There was no headache, except from Meredith constantly warning me to keep my head down.

I tried to quiet my mind and ignore thoughts about the future. Each time I saw hope lingering, I was tempted to push the door closed. Of course I wanted to allow, even invite, hope in, but I did not trust that emotion. Deterioration was all I had known. My ability to find faith in the future still was negligible. Decades of disappointment had made it all but impossible to allow myself to hope for something better. Self-protection is a powerful instinct. As much as I trusted the Tisch team, I had little faith in my body, a machine that had betrayed me too many times.

CHAPTER 17

Star and Crescent

I t was time for me to stop simply researching organized religions and figure out what the faithful know that I had been missing. During a conversation in Dr. Sadiq's private office one afternoon, I reminded him of my interest in attending Friday prayers with him. He already had agreed to take me to the service, but I had not followed up. "Just tell me when you want to go," Sadiq said with no hesitation. How about next week? I suggested. Fine.

The prospect of spending time in a church or synagogue had no appeal for me. I had fled those houses of worship decades ago. Attending Friday prayers was different. On Friday afternoon the following week, Sadiq and I walked into the nondescript side entrance of the Church of Saint Paul the Apostle, a grand Roman Catholic church on Manhattan's West Side. The structure brought elegance to a once dirty, dicey neighborhood known as Hell's Kitchen. Paulist fathers had built this imposing, Gothic fortress in 1858.

Catholicism and Islam may seem a strange fit, but this is New York, where real estate is expensive, and institutions of faith are known to reach out to each other when space to worship is needed. As he had told me, Sadiq had approached the church about the possibility of holding Friday prayers there more than five years earlier.

The Muslim group Sadiq had put together had outgrown the space they were using in a small basement room at St. Luke's–Roosevelt Hospital, where he ran the MS care unit. Since St. Paul's was just a short walk from Sadiq's office, this church offered the perfect solution.

Sadiq told me that when he went to church officials to make the request, he wore a jacket and tie but explained that the men and women who would be coming to the service would not be dressed the same way. They would be individuals of modest means, immigrant cabdrivers based in the area, and laborers of various kinds. Many had come from Senegal and Mali and other Muslim countries. They were folks who wanted to take a short break from their work and come together to pray.

"Most of them will look very suspicious to you, and you will be afraid that maybe they are terrorists," he had told church officials. "But they are peaceful, and you will have nothing to worry about." The answer came quickly. Yes.

Paulists are known for charting their own course, even opening their arms to gay and lesbian Catholics and reaching out to women who have undergone abortions. The fact that they opened their doors to a Muslim group in search of a venue to meet and pray is very much part of their tradition of independence.

We walked into the church on that cold, windy day, and I stood and watched the worshippers gradually enter the building. They were primarily Africans, speaking unfamiliar languages in quiet, respectful tones. All wore simple clothes. They seemed subdued and serious.

Sadiq and I made our way upstairs to the room set aside for the service. A plain cardboard box had been placed on a folding chair at the door. Participants left a dollar or two if they could as they filed in, a gesture of thanks to the church.

Everyone removed their shoes and left them at the entrance to the prayer space as they went into the room. Dirt is not to be tracked into the House of Allah. The ritual washing of hands, feet, and face that happens before a typical Muslim service was not possible because of a lack of facilities.

Sadiq touched my arm and told me I didn't have to remove my shoes. He knows I cannot walk without shoes because my toes curl under my feet. Sadiq guided me to a folding chair propped against a wall. I wished I could join the others as they took to the floor to sit to pray, but that was not an option for me. Once I am horizontal on the floor, I am there for an extended visit. Besides, I would not have followed the others as they sat, stood, and laid flat, their foreheads touching the floor during the service. I am not a Muslim, and others might have been offended if I had tried to mimic their moves. I was determined to show respect.

While waiting for the service to begin, I looked around at the space. The room had seemed large when we walked in, but that changed as worshippers arrived in groups. I had wondered how others would react to me. I had the only white face in the space. The attendees were warm and welcoming, some approaching me to shake my hand before the service. I was totally comfortable.

The service was more muted than I had expected. There were the ritual prayers, most in Arabic. There was no singing, unlike in Jewish and Christian services. A soft-spoken young Yemeni physician named Marwan Alahiri, who is applying for a residency in neurology in the United States, offered the sermon. Marwan is a serious student of Islam who has memorized the Quran. The sermon was vehemently anti-violence. Marwan's tone was unyielding. Though much of the service had been in Arabic, Marwan delivered the sermon in clear English.

For a while I lost sight of Sadiq in the sea of prostrate bodies. Following the service, he resurfaced and introduced me to Marwan, who listened attentively as I told him about this research into hope and what I wanted to accomplish. Marwan is a small man with a large heart who seemed to genuinely care about the health issues that had motivated me to embark on this investigation of hope.

Unlike most of the worshippers, who appeared to be from working-class backgrounds, Marwan was polished, even scholarly. He made clear he would be happy to sit down and talk about the role of hope in his faith. We agreed to meet the following week at the Tisch center, where he works in Sadiq's lab.

The three of us exited the church together that afternoon, just a few New Yorkers ambling up Tenth Avenue, huddled against the wind and shooting the breeze. We had left our serious sides at the church door. I thought of how often religion becomes a wedge, separating us from one another. Yet I felt a real connection with these men.

The next week I arrived at the Tisch center to take Marwan up on his offer to talk. The staff shot me looks, wondering why I was there without an appointment. I mumbled something, offering a nonanswer. Why would I be visiting Marwan? I could not think of how to explain it, since I was not sure if anyone in the office even knew about Friday prayers.

I looked for Marwan, and as I was rounding the corner of one of the many corridors in the sprawling Tisch center, there he was. We exchanged smiles, shook hands, and ducked into the empty infusion suite, around the corner from the lab. Marwan asked me to tell him more about what I thought he could offer. Soon he was talking about the Quran and hope, exactly what I was there to hear.

The subject seemed so complicated to me. For starters, I needed a primer in Marwan's religion, one that was short, sweet, and accessible. When I asked Marwan what Islam teaches about hope, he found a passage in the Quran that he thought would answer my question.

"Whosoever fears Allah . . . He will make a way for him to get out from every difficulty. And He will provide for him from sources he could never imagine." (Quran 65:2–3) "Isn't that what hope is all about?" Marwan asked. He seemed to think this passage would be instructive to me. It was not.

Doesn't this mean you have to be a follower of Allah to find hope? I asked. "No," Marwan answered. "That is a general principle for everybody. It's a fact of life." It sounded to me as though hope comes from belief in Allah, I countered. In this and any number of other verses from the Quran, it seems clear that divine benevolence goes only to those who love or fear Allah. What about the rest of us?

Marwan went on: "If you read the Quran, you will see many verses inspiring people not to lose hope." But how? I wanted to know. If you are sick or starving or in terrible danger, and you don't believe in Allah, what makes it possible to keep hoping? "The word *patience* is mentioned in the Quran more than ninety times," Marwan counseled. "We have to learn patience."

I have been hearing that word from doctors forever. I imagine most of us who grapple with serious sickness become impatient with the call for patience. Marwan was not giving up. The Quran speaks to that frustration, he told me. He was aware of my medical history and understood why I sounded exasperated. He quoted a passage that he thought would help put the call for patience into context.

"Do you think that you will enter paradise without such trials as came to those who passed away before you? They experienced suffering and adversity and were so shaken in spirit that even the Prophet and the faithful who were with him cried, 'When will Allah's help come.' Ah, verily the help of Allah is near." (Quran 2:214)

We were back to Allah and to my feeling that in Islam, as in other faiths, the goodies are reserved for believers. No, Marwan said, and quoted yet another passage he thought would interest me. Or shut me up. "So, verily, with every difficulty, there is ease: Verily with every difficulty there is relief." (Quran 94:5–6)

If only I could believe that, but I am a tough customer when it comes to believing in the possibility of relief, since I have found so little over the years. Marwan went home that day without quite convincing me. The last passage he had quoted did stay with me, and I was curious about how he thought it might apply to coping with a serious illness.

When I emailed Marwan to ask, he responded: "This verse is part of a chapter of the Quran revealed when difficulties were weighing the Prophet Muhammad down and causing him distress. The words of God comforted and reassured him. Life is not either all good or all bad . . . God reminds us that with hardship comes ease. Hardship is never absolute."

That is a nice thought, I replied, but I never have seen

evidence that good follows bad. In the medical mayhem that has become my life, bad only seems to lead to worse. Such is the nature of a series of illnesses that feed off one another. Many systems in the body can falter. Many are interdependent. Are bad and good really cyclical? I just do not think so.

"The verse does not mean after the bad times come good times," Marwan explained. "Saying that with hardship comes ease means that there is always something to be grateful for. God gives us strength and patience." That gratitude is an article of faith, a core belief. Neither Sadiq nor Marwan seem prone to doubt or skepticism. They are smart men, indeed wise, who happen to be absolute believers. They are typical of the 84 percent of Muslims who say they are absolutely certain that God exists, a considerably higher percentage than among Christians or Jews.

Sadiq also showed patience with my endless questions. During one of my later visits to his office, I asked him whether he thought nonbelievers would be cut off from reaping the rewards of a good life. As always, Sadiq had an answer. "While alive, everyone is under the mercy and blessing of Allah, whether you believe in his existence or not. After death, only Allah is the judge and sole jury of whether you are a Muslim or not." In my book, that is not due process.

As a non-Muslim, I doubt I can count on Allah's mercy. And that leads me to yet another question. How can Allah or Jehovah, Yahweh or whatever god one worships, sit in judgment of someone of another faith? Or none at all? Am I wrong?

One day I told Sadiq that I didn't understand what drives a person to worship. What is the payoff for prayer? I asked. "I feel like I am reaching my creator in some way," he answered, showing his usual forbearance. "I get an inner strength and an energy." Sadiq paused. "It makes me aware of my connection to God. I feel like I am a better person and a stronger person. The connection gives me hope."

Sadiq is all-in. I know Christians and Jews who half-worship their god. They attend services a few times a year, mostly on predictable holidays. Otherwise they pack up religion and save it for a rainy day. For the observant Muslims I met, faith seems to be a way of life. Believers take a large view of faith and build it into their daily existence. For them, the currency of the realm is not hope but assumption. Their questions have been answered.

From what Sadiq said, Islam provides what he called a recipe for making this connection. "In the search for God, you follow the recipe," he told me, "which means, in my case, you fast two days a week and pray up to six or seven times per day."

Islam seems to be highly doctrinal. The Quran comes across as black and white. And I am uncomfortable with orthodoxy in any form. In Christianity, *orthodoxy* means, "conforming to the Christian faith as represented in the creeds of the early Church." I escaped Sunday school decades ago and never had a wish to conform to anything. Why start now?

The idea that hope is owned exclusively by the faithful is

one reason so many of us seeking spiritual self-determination find organized religion stifling. I believe hope is a very personal idea that has to grow from within. The search for hope is served by open minds and the willingness to challenge conventional thinking.

CHAPTER 18

Blindsided, Again

On a frigid night in late March 2014, Meredith and I had separate commitments in the city. I arrived home first. As I got out of the car to walk into the house, I began to hyperventilate fiercely. By the time I reached the front door, I thought I was going to collapse. I made it to the kitchen and rested. I did not know what was going on, but, true to form, I decided it was nothing to be concerned about.

When I went upstairs, I couldn't breathe again. I barely made it to the bedroom. Meredith happened to call at that moment. I told her what was going on, adding that I was not worried. Meredith took her cues from me, and the subject was dropped.

A week went by with no further episodes. That cold night was pretty much forgotten. On Saturday evening, we were expecting friends to stop by for an early drink. I stepped out of the shower, donned jeans and a T-shirt, and went through the closet, looking for my well-worn boat shoes. By now they were held together with gaffer's tape. I should have been embarrassed to be seen in those ugly shoes, but at our house, dressing up can mean dressing down.

I sat on the edge of the bed and put on my left shoe. When I tried to slip on the right shoe, I could not get my foot into it. No matter how much I pushed and pulled, the shoe would not go on. This was not right. These were old stretched-out shoes. They were so loose that sometimes I had trouble keeping them on my feet.

Strange, I thought. With one shoe on and the other in my hand, I hobbled into my study, where there was more light and I could see what I was doing. I sat at my desk and tried once more. Again, the shoe would not go on. Finally, I leaned over to try to figure out what the problem was. I had to get my eyes close to the floor because my vision is so bad.

My foot was huge. I yelled to Meredith, asking her to come upstairs and take a quick look. She squinted and was taken aback.

"My foot is as large as Cleveland," I said quietly. I knew something was very wrong. "Your big toenail is turning black," Meredith told me.

I sat motionless, unsure of what to do or who to contact. Saturday night is not the optimal time to find a doctor and ask a question. We sat in silence. I assumed Sadiq would be in his office. He always is. I called his cell, even though I figured a swollen foot had nothing to do with a stem cell infusion. I thought he might have some advice anyway. He did. "Hang up the phone right now and get to an emergency room," he said with unusual urgency in his voice. "I think you have a blood clot."

Do I really need to do that? I asked myself. I could just shrug off the whole thing and go sit by the fire and wait for our friends to arrive. That was tempting on this cold, damp evening. Meredith and I sat upstairs for a moment and stared at each other.

I did give a passing thought to the time when another doctor had told me I should go for my first colonoscopy. I came close to ignoring him. When I went ahead with the procedure, the gastroenterologist discovered a malignant polyp. Two bouts of colon cancer later, I was still alive, and I figured it was because I had followed doctor's orders. My record on that score was not always so good.

I decided to again be a grown-up. If I hadn't, Meredith would have dragged me to a hospital against my will anyway. We got in the car and drove to a small hospital only a mile from home. I had called our friends to tell them what was happening. I told them I was sure we'd see them in an hour.

They later told me I was strangely calm on the phone. *Oblivious* is a better word. I did think we would soon get to the bottom of this and salvage the evening, which was my primary focus. Sadiq's ominous tone was just not computing for me, even though I never had heard him speak that way.

The ER seemed empty. We live in a quiet suburban area where weekend emergencies are infrequent. When I showed the attending doctor my foot, he did not have any visible reaction, but he quickly ordered a series of tests, including a chest X-ray, a Doppler ultrasound scan of my leg, and a CT scan.

First came the ultrasound. An orderly put me into a wheelchair and delivered me to the radiology department, where there was a wait because the technician who would perform the test had to come in from a neighboring town. Within minutes of her arrival, she was running the wand up and down both legs. She announced, and repeated several times, that she was not allowed to tell me what she was seeing. Strange, I thought, since I was not asking.

The attending doctor addressed the results of the leg scan immediately after I returned to the ER. "You have a sizable blood clot in your right leg." I stared at him in silence. "Actually, it extends from your ankle almost to your knee." I was speechless. Meredith did not react. "We need to start you on blood thinners immediately."

What seemed to concern the doctor was the size of the clot. "We can't fool around with this," he said. I just nodded, unable to say anything. This was not what I had bargained for, even though it was exactly what Sadiq had predicted on the phone. My pulse quickened as I began to think things were getting out of hand.

Before I knew what was happening, an IV line was inserted into my arm and an infusion of heparin, a blood thinner commonly used to treat clots, was started. The ER staff explained it was important that I remain in the hospital overnight to allow the drug to do its work.

Damn, I thought. So much for my new lease on life with the stem cells. I had survived cancer and sworn never to spend another night in any hospital on this planet. A lot of bad memories were stored in my head. I did not want to relive them. At the very least, this was not how I wanted to spend my Saturday night.

I knew heparin was a routine blood-clot treatment, and for some reason that kept me from being particularly alarmed. I already was establishing emotional distance from the problem. I was practiced at that. It was as if we were there to deal with someone else's swollen foot.

All I wanted was to go home. I knew that impulse was childlike, but I did not care. At the moment, my thumb was in my mouth. I took it out just long enough to reluctantly agree that, yes, it probably was a good idea for me to stay where nurses could monitor the blood thinner.

After the CT scan, when Meredith and I were alone in my room, we agreed that we did not know what to make of life's new wrinkle. I felt I had been ambushed, but I was pretty sure I would survive the clot. I had no basis for that optimistic attitude, but it felt reassuring.

Just as we were beginning to calm down from the urgency

of the last few hours and trying to focus on the next steps, a nurse hurried into the room. I looked at her, saw the expression on her face, and before she even said a word felt the hair on the back of my neck stand on end.

"You have to get out of here," she announced. "A piece of the clot broke off and is in your pulmonary artery between your heart and lungs. This is dangerous." Electricity shot through my body. "You have to get to a hospital that has an intensive care unit," she told us. "Ours closed years ago."

And with that, she was gone. No doctor showed up to see me. No administrator came to help us coordinate my transfer to another hospital. This was a small place in a suburban town on a dreary Saturday night. Very few doctors and nurses were around. We were on our own.

The silence the nurse left behind was deafening. Meredith and I looked at each other for a long moment, attempting to process what we had just heard. Then we got down to business and started figuring out what our options were. Once we realized we were in charge, we knew we needed to think fast and make decisions, unfortunately on the basis of very little information.

Did I have to find a new hospital at this very moment? I did not have a clue, but an ambulance ride into New York seemed to be in my near future. We figured only major medical centers could handle this kind of emergency. Mount Sinai Hospital was the one place where I had a relationship.

I had been on the board of the MS center there and had been awarded an honorary degree from its medical school. But when a nurse called to check the availability at Mount Sinai, she was told they were full. We did not know what to do. Meredith then called a friend of ours who is on the board of trustees there. He came through for us. I wondered how anybody without connections survived the medical jungles.

In the early afternoon the following day, I was wheeled from the ambulance onto ramps and whisked up elevators into Mount Sinai. We crashed through the double doors of the intensive care unit. A full crew was waiting for me there. This was the real thing.

From the moment I entered that big-city ICU, there was a total loss of control. When I looked around, the ICU seemed to go on forever and hold an endless number of beds, all with curtains closed around them. The unrelenting sound of muffled voices mixed with every electronic sound possible became the white noise of the ICU. And it did not stop.

Loud staccato shouts cut through the space. Nobody seemed to talk at a normal volume. Lights always were flashing or flickering. People rushed about. The place was controlled chaos. Now, my memory may be embellished by fear. Memory, in moments of high stress, can be tricky.

I was immediately taken to a bed, where the nurses pulled off my street clothes and put me into gowns. The room was cold, but they surrounded me with warm blankets. One nurse rubbed me with fragrant oils. It felt as if they were preparing my body for burial.

I kept shaking my head in disbelief, as if I had wandered into someone else's nightmare. Yet I was certain I was awake, eliminating the enticing possibility that this was all a dream that would end as soon as I opened my clenched eyes.

Shortly after I arrived, a group of young doctors hooked me up to multiple machines making strange noises. My veins were so deflated that the chief resident decided to put a port into my neck to insert the IV. There were so many people around, coming and going, doing so many things to me seemingly all at the same time. I had no idea what was happening.

I was dazed by the amount of activity, groggy beyond sleep deprivation, and completely disoriented. My senses were heightened. It felt as if I had smoked too much weed in a crowd. The ICU was jammed and getting more so by the hour. As stretchers came and went, sounds of urgency echoed through the open space. Dozens of dramas were playing out on this crowded stage.

At one point in these first hours, a lung specialist came to see me. When he asked about my recent medical history, I casually mentioned the previous week's episode of hyperventilation, attributing it to the oral steroid I had been taking. The pulmonologist just stared at me.

"That was the clot moving to your lungs," he told me. "It sat there for eight days. You have a pulmonary embolism and are lucky to be alive." It was as though he was scolding me for my stupidity. I have never had a pulmonary embolism before, I thought. I will know better next time.

The prospect of there being a next time was precisely what worried the doctors. It worried me too. There was a time bomb in my body. The clot in my leg was large, and it was sobering to recognize how fortunate I was to be breathing. I had long ago convinced myself I was staying at least one step ahead of the MS and cancer that stalked me. I had not been cocky, but I was confident I was winning.

Now this. I was flirting with a total loss. A near-death moment lasts a lifetime. I wondered if I would move past the what-ifs and just allow myself to be glad I was still around. But of course, I did not know whether the crisis was over.

The pulmonologist had talked to Meredith after seeing me and told her that this could go either way. The first forty-eight hours would be critical. I was in the fight of my life, but I did not fully appreciate that until later, because Meredith discreetly forgot to mention this conversation to me until the crisis really had passed.

Day melted into night. There was no natural light to signal the change. When I tried to sleep, I discovered that nodding off is all anyone can expect in an intensive care unit. Sustained sleep is impossible. At best, patients slip in and out of consciousness in the midst of the frenzy of activity and bright lights, crazy noise levels, and general mayhem. Sleep happens only when exhaustion takes over. Battlefields offer no comfortable hotel rooms. Meredith spent most of her time by my bed, sleeping as little as I did.

Twenty-four hours after I was admitted, an interventional radiologist stood over me in a cramped space in the basement. This was a specialty that was new to me. According to a Johns Hopkins website, "Interventional radiology is a medical sub-specialty of radiology, utilizing minimally-invasive image-guided procedures to diagnose and treat diseases in nearly every organ system." Monitors flickered as the doctor squinted, staring intently at the image of my torso.

I liked this guy. He actually talked to me, explaining exactly what he was about to do. He would be inserting a filter into a vein in my groin and threading it up into my abdominal cavity, where it would be opened. The filter is known as an umbrella and is designed to catch any future clots before they can do damage to vital organs. The procedure was painless.

The pulmonologist explained that after a few months I would have to decide if I wanted to keep the filter in place. Me? I had to decide? I also had to make a decision whether or not to stay on a blood thinner. I said yes to both. The pulmonologist told me, "Your clot is slowly shrinking because of the blood thinners, but you still have a large clot in your leg. Another piece could break off and do terrible damage." In other words, it would kill me.

In the first days of my stay in ICU, Meredith stayed in

touch with Sadiq, keeping him abreast of developments. Both of us believed he had saved my life with his decisive and firm advice to go to an emergency room immediately. Meredith told me Sadiq wanted to know everything that was happening. Since he had no connection to Mount Sinai, he could not follow my progress in person, but his concern and interest made me feel his presence. That meant a lot to me at a time when I felt very fragile.

How close I had come to leaving this life was not lost on me. For the eight days after the clot had moved to my chest, I was on a high wire without knowing it. I remained in the ICU for several long days and nights. The IV blood thinners continued as the doctors waited and watched, monitoring the clot in my leg until they saw it was not moving. It had shrunk enough that I was no longer in imminent danger. When I finally was moved to a private room, it was as if I had been sprung from prison. This confirmed what I suspected: I was going to survive.

We had urged our kids not to make the trip home during the blood-clot scare. Ben was living in Shanghai at the time. Lily was still at college in Chicago. And Gabe was working as a television reporter in Spokane. There was nothing they could do for me, and it seemed unnecessary to disrupt their lives. Gabe decided to take matters into his own hands. He just showed up at the hospital one day.

Once I had stabilized, Gabe and Meredith were ready to

take me home. Because of my nagging skin condition, how-ever, the doctors were not yet willing to release me. I still itched like crazy. So it came as a relief when I was told that Mark Lebwohl, the chief of the Department of Dermatology, would be coming to see me. I was pleased the pulmonary embolism was no longer an issue, equally pleased that at last I was to be seen by someone who might be able to do some-thing about the horrible skin condition that had been wearing me down for months.

Dr. Lebwohl unleashed his army of dermatology residents on me. He finally delivered his diagnosis. "You have erythro-dermic psoriasis," he told me. Great. This was another in-flammatory autoimmune disease, just like MS. I was slightly schooled in the genetic connections between certain diseases. I was certain this was no coincidence. Later I asked a Harvard geneticist if he agreed. "Yes," he answered, "but I couldn't prove it."

I had no reason to doubt Lebwohl's diagnosis. The man had authored a respected textbook on psoriasis and is an ex-pert on the subject. He began treating me with a slow-acting drug that he said would eventually do the job, though I would probably lose a lot of hair. I did not care about that, but I did care that I had another disease to joust with.

My week of living dangerously was coming to an end. It was time to check out of the hospital and check back into my life. The doctors had kept me alive, and I was grateful. I did not need to be told twice to go home to my own bed. But even though I was released from the hospital, I came to realize that you really cannot go home again.

The man who left Mount Sinai was a different person from the guy who had showed up in his local ER suddenly one Saturday evening. I was crisis-free, and relieved. But I was a deflated balloon and almost out of gas. If there is a god, I thought, He was raising a middle finger to me. Of course, that gesture was absolutely reciprocal.

When I was home again, I sat in silence. I hung out in the family room, clinging to the safety of sitting in my ratty old chair, torn up by too many cats for too long. I breathed easier just being back in my own house, still stunned by my recent foray into New York City. I had traveled far in one week. I reread Virginia Woolf's 1926 essay "On Being Ill." "How astonishing, when the lights of health go down, the undiscovered countries that are then disclosed, what wastes and deserts of the soul."

Seven days had seemed to last a lifetime. There was no map for the trip I had taken. The journey had left me dazed and disoriented, searching for an explanation that did not seem to exist. I longed for clarity and closure but was stuck on the vision of lying lifeless on the floor of my bedroom, dropped by a blood clot in my lungs.

I needed answers, not more questions. And yet, not long after I escaped the hospital, there was one more ailment I had to deal with. I had started to notice painful sores on my chest. I called my internist in New York and described them. "It sounds like shingles," he said.

No.

I like my internist. He knew I did not want to go back to the city to visit his office after having just left. He suggested having Meredith take a few photos of my chest and emailing them to him. We did that and he got back to me very quickly. He had looked at the photos and showed them to a dermatologist. The diagnosis was confirmed. Shingles. Are you freaking kidding me? Piling on draws a penalty in football, but I heard no whistles blow. I did not react. My tank was empty.

I could see nothing but a vast black hole, an emptiness that extended as far as the eye could see. I feared I was falling into that space. Not only was there no map to guide me; there seemed to be no road. When I was young, I knew I had a destination. It was not always visible, but I trusted it was there. My direction was true. Faith in my future was strong. I had strength that carried me a great distance. My confidence in myself was mighty. Isn't that what hope is?

Over the years the road forked, diverging again and again. From time to time the trip grew perilous. Serious sickness kept ambushing me, and I often felt lost. I always found my way back, but sometimes I was gone so long that when I returned, home was a different place.

This time I felt I no longer knew the way back. The loss of hope was quick but familiar. The emotional pain felt new. I was struggling to stand, both literally and figuratively. I moped around the house for months, as dazed as a punch-drunk boxer. Every hint of hope was gone, replaced by nothing. I was spent, emotionally incapacitated. I was not angry, just running on fumes. This went beyond the usual hope vacuum to a feeling of genuine loss.

I tried to change my daily routine. I believed the clots had been caused by too much time sitting in the same position at the computer. Healthy people move their legs around when they sit. Because of the MS, I have a right foot that is essentially a dead weight. My legs do not shift when I am sitting.

My hands move across a keyboard, but my feet remain frozen beneath me. I knew I needed to make changes to my sedentary life and spend more time on my feet. I drank more water, necessitating an increased number of trips to the bathroom. That meant time on my feet. I figured every little bit helped.

I was scheduled for my second stem cell infusion in late August. Procedurally, this one was like the first, but it was markedly different in that the infusion came and went with no particular hopes or expectations. The procedure was completely uneventful. The infusion process took the same amount of time, fifteen minutes or so, and was followed by the same three hours of boredom, lying prone and taking in the IV antibiotics.

I really did try to be hopeful that I might see some improvement. There had been nothing to show from the first go-round, even though Sadiq had warned me this might be the case. I needed movement in the right direction. So much had gone wrong since the first infusion. I felt it was time for something to go right.

I worried that my various medical crises might be sabotaging the good work of the millions of stem cells now swimming in my spine. Dr. Sadiq tried to be reassuring, but he could not talk me out of my concern. This therapy is new. No one knows. We were pioneers heading into a vast stretch of new territory. We do know what can happen to pioneers moving across rugged terrain.

I still like being a pioneer, and even with my frustration, I knew the stem cell experiment held all kinds of possibilities. Still, I wondered if my age was an issue here. Does a guy in his midsixties have the same potential to respond as a younger person? Or is he likely to collapse on the prairie, another pioneer unable to make it to the promised land?

We will find out. In any case, as far as I am concerned, this experiment is as much for my children as it is for me. I am the third generation in my family to be hit by MS. I hope there never will be a fourth. If the worst does happen, I want a revolutionary therapy ready and waiting, ammunition to spare the next generation. That is the fiercest hope I know.

A few weeks after the second infusion, Meredith and I took Lily to a restaurant in town for a farewell dinner. She had come home for summer vacation and was driving back to

Chicago early the next morning to begin her senior year in college. I could not process the idea that our little girl was almost ready to go out into the world. We ordered drinks and made a toast. We wanted to wish her a safe trip.

Before our food arrived, I began to feel weak. It came on gradually. In the next forty-five minutes, I started nodding off. I realized I was disconnected from the once bubbly, now muted conversation. There were moments when my head hung so low it almost rested on the table. I hadn't finished that one drink, so I couldn't have been reacting to the alcohol. Meredith and Lily noticed I was struggling and wanted to leave. I insisted I was okay, and besides, we still hadn't gotten our dinners.

By the time the waiter served us, I was too out of it to eat. Meredith and Lily picked at their food. We sat in silence. When we did stand to leave, I moved unsteadily toward the door. I could go no farther. While Lily went to get the car, the proprietor and a few of his buddies managed to maneuver me down three steep steps to the street. When Lily pulled up, I could see tears rolling down her cheeks. I sat in the front seat next to her but could not bring myself to look at her. Another evening ruined by this cursed disease, was all I could think. I could not stand making Lily cry.

Fuck this trial, I silently screamed.

CHAPTER 19

Psychology and Biology of Hope

I n this competitive world, big hopes call for smart strategies. According to an article in *Psychology Today*, "Talent, skill, ability—whatever you want to call it—will not get you there . . . A wealth of psychological research over the past few decades show loud and clear that it's the psychological *vehicles* that really get you there." Athletes are agents of big business, but they play on fields of dreams. In the end, sports stars are powered by hope and determination. So, too, are fans, and fans matter because the energy in the stands can fuel the action on the field.

In 2016, Chicago was taken over by hope for one long summer, and many could not let go. Residents and visitors wrote notes to relatives and friends, departed Cubs fans who did not live to witness baseball history. That practice began as the season progressed, and the team closed in on the title. Messages were scrawled in chalk on a brick wall in the bleachers. After the series, fans climbed ladders and stood on accommodating shoulders to find blank spaces to write to loved ones.

Dr. Kenneth Ravizza is a top sports psychologist who has worked with U.S. Olympians and teams such as the New York Jets as well as college teams such as the University of Nebraska Cornhuskers. Ken and I went to high school together. Ken was a star athlete while I was busy getting thrown off the soccer team for drinking beer. I would be suspended from school later that year, though I really cannot remember why. I was a troublemaker and a malcontent, assuring my future career in the news business.

Ken and I had lost touch years ago. We reconnected at a class reunion in 2003. Each of us had to pass up our fiftieth high school reunion in 2016 because Ken was at the World Series as an integral part of the Chicago Cubs organization and I was busy chasing hope.

In the 2016 season, the Chicago Cubs were hot. So were Cubs loyalists. The spark missing for more than a century had been ignited. The Cubs and their fans became partners, and Chicago became a city of hope. The long-suffering fan base became part of the winning equation, with the energy in the bleachers fused with what was happening on the field.

I wanted to talk to Ken about it, so I reached him at his home on the West Coast, where he had been on the faculty of California State University Fullerton until his retirement in

2015. When we talked, Ken made it clear that he does not speak for the Cubs organization, only for himself. Perfect, I answered. I want to know what you think.

"I think the mental game is a big part of baseball," Ken began. "Under pressure, a player's skills get better or they get worse." Major League Baseball is a high-stakes game for everyone on the field, and the pressure can result in enormous amounts of stress. Learning how to handle pressure is critical. Ken pointed out that the all-powerful self-assured athlete is a mythological character. "Confidence is very fragile with elite athletes. They have swagger on TV. They have all that stuff. In reality, they are human beings like all of us, and their confidence wavers." Ravizza understands that athletes fear that their game will suffer if there are any cracks in their armor.

Ken works hard to keep his players feeling good, though he knows that, for players, staying focused and sure of themselves 100 percent of the time just is not possible. "Your belief in yourself comes and goes over the duration of the season."

Ken tries to bring a real-world approach to his work with his players, teaching them that in times of uncertainty and anxiety, they can soldier on past any feelings of self-doubt. "Part of the mental game is getting the guys to believe that they don't have to feel totally confident all the time. If they do the preparation, they don't have to feel good to do well. That is a big part of our mental skills program."

Ravizza takes on the long season one pitch at a time. "I tell a pitcher, before you make the pitch, you have to have conviction. You have to commit to what you are about to do. You are better off with one hundred percent conviction on the wrong pitch than eighty percent on the right pitch." Whether a player is a batter fighting a strong opposing pitcher or a fan struggling with a dangerous disease, I believe hope feeds the conviction that winning is possible.

Ken, however, does not see conviction and hope as the same thing. "If the guy is hoping he's going to execute the pitch, that ain't going to work. You can't just be hoping and praying. You have to bring conviction to what you are doing." In my mind, it is not a question of either-or. Conviction implies strength, as if a result can be willed into being. It is all a mind game, and I am convinced hope must creep into a player's head.

"Hope is survival," Ken said. "And that is as primal as it gets. The whole body is wired for hope." There was a momentary silence before I realized Ken was addressing my battles, not telling me about sending a message to his players. "That is what motivates us to do anything." Perhaps players and patients have a lot in common.

The hope I imagine is not passive. It is not as simple as "just hoping and praying." Hope requires action. It takes hard work, mental flexibility, a willingness to keep one's eye on the prize. People have to continually adjust their understanding of just what the prize is.

I play in a different arena from any baseball player. For me, the prize is protecting, even recovering my health. I think of my drive to overcome my many maladies. I am determined to up my batting average and beat them, though I realize that may not even be possible. I have enough of a competitive spirit that I continue to take the field, and my family and friends are in the stands.

If hope has the power to keep us going, how do we explain its work in the body? Is hope simply a mind game, or does hope play out in some mysterious way physically? My bottom-line question was simple: Can hope be self-fulfilling?

I had a chance to find out more about how hope could manifest physiologically when Meredith and I went to Boston on a chilly day in October 2016. We were attending the opening of the new Building for Transformative Medicine at Brigham and Women's Hospital, which houses the new Institute for the Neurosciences. The Brigham, as the place is commonly called, is one of the sixteen hospitals and research centers affiliated with Harvard Medical School.

There was a homecoming quality for me on this day. I had warm memories of my work on the advisory council of the Harvard NeuroDiscovery Center. A number of physician-scientists I knew from my time there now were part of the fledgling institute at the Brigham.

I am also on the advisory council of the new Brigham

Institute. Meredith sits on the advisory board of the Ann Romney Center for Neurologic Diseases, which is part of the institute. She had been asked to interview three prominent physicians on this day at a gathering of donors and guests. This would be the first public event in the new building, and I was pleased to cross paths again with friends and acquaintances.

We were milling around a large sitting area, saying hello and being introduced to new people before the program began. I sat in a comfortable chair and chatted with various folks. After a while, Dr. Martin Samuels ambled over and sat at my side. This tall, thin seventy-two-year-old physician is chairman of neurology at the Brigham and directs the Institute for the Neurosciences.

I had been meeting informally with Marty for more than a year, discussing plans for the new institute and trading ideas. Physicians in leadership positions at Harvard frequently seek counsel from individuals from a variety of backgrounds. When I told him of my questions about hope, he said he thought he could make a contribution. Marty talked quickly because people were beginning to move to the designated space for the event.

I wasn't able to catch everything he said in that noisy room. I would have loved to have taken notes, but I had nothing to write with and have pretty much lost the ability even to hold a pen. MS is the gift that keeps on giving. I thought I remembered the good doctor use the words *voodoo death* in our brief conversation. Could I have heard that correctly? We made our way to the ceremony and lost track of each other in the crowd. I was left wondering what he could have possibly meant.

A few months later, I joined Marty in his old office for coffee. The Brigham sits across the street from Harvard Medical School, an elegant fortress in look and feel. To reach Marty's office required going down endless corridors and around corners, a long-enough hike that I had to use a wheelchair to get there.

Marty picked up our conversation about hope, describing a patient he had treated during his residency at Boston City Hospital. The patient had suffered a spontaneous hemorrhage in his brain, which left him unconscious.

The man also had a very abnormal cardiogram, a measure of heart function. Marty told me he had been intrigued by the fact that this man was afflicted by both conditions. The significance of the apparent coincidence was lost on me, but Marty had the sense this was not a coincidence at all, that there was a link between the two. The young doctor decided to figure this out.

"None of the senior residents knew how the brain could have caused the heart to malfunction. That was the single case that got me turned on to this connection between the nervous system and the heart." Marty believes he later solved the mystery. Following the brain event, the man had regained consciousness, and it became clear he had lost hope.

Marty continued, "This is the mirror image of what you are writing about. It is the absence of hope, the disappearance of hope, and its deleterious effect." The doctor was on a roll. "This answers the question, Does hope help? There is no question. The negative effect of hopelessness is backed up by a combination of empirical evidence and anecdote."

Dr. Samuels presented his case in greater detail when he and I met again in late 2016 at the Library Hotel in New York. He and his wife, Susan Pioli, a longtime medical publisher, joined me for coffee. Marty carried his laptop. He had prepared a presentation to explain the negative power of hopelessness and how it can affect the body. We moved to a large table, and Marty set up the visual presentation.

He began with a display of old photos. The first was a vintage image of Walter Bradford Cannon, one of America's leading early-twentieth-century physiologists. Born in 1871 and educated at Harvard Medical School, Cannon was a pioneer in understanding the influence of emotion on body function.

"Cannon conceptualized the fight-or-flight dynamic, which argues that when an animal is under a life-threatening stressor, there is a system within the brain that causes the secretion of a hormone, which we call adrenaline." Adrenaline causes the heart to beat faster, the blood to be transferred from the gut to the brain, and the pupils to dilate for better vision. These reactions are part of what Cannon called the sympathetic nervous system, which exercises control over blood flow and the internal organs of the body.

In 1942, Cannon published a paper titled "'Voodoo' Death." I sat up straight. I had not imagined the phrase after all. "Cannon recounted numerous reports of people in South America, Africa, and elsewhere who had been put under spells or curses and inexplicably died."

Dr. Cannon tracked down trained observers who had witnessed these deaths to see if they could confirm the accuracy of the reports. They did. There seemed to be no observable cause of death and no underlying illness, no secret poisoning and nothing to explain what had happened.

As Marty described Cannon's investigation, the narrative took on the feeling of a murder mystery. Who or what had killed these people? What Cannon wondered was "whether an ominous and persistent state of fear can end the life of a man." If so, what was the physiological basis for such a death?

Cannon decided it was because of the "persistent excessive activity" of the sympathetic nervous system. A person who believes himself under a curse, a situation over which he has no control and in which he has no chance of possible survival, will be terrified. Marty paused for emphasis. "Talk about lack of hope. There it is."

The historic, if anecdotal, evidence corroborating the

effect of this powerful emotion on the body is spellbinding, he went on. It appears as early as the New Testament. In Acts 5:1–10, a man named Ananias and his wife, Sapphira, sold a piece of property. Though Ananias wanted it to appear that he was giving all the proceeds of the sale to the apostle Peter, he brought only part of the money to him and kept the rest for himself. Peter asked Ananias how Satan had so filled his heart that he would lie to the Holy Spirit. "You have not lied just to human beings," Peter said, "but to God." When Ananias heard this, he fell down and died.

Hours later, Sapphira returned and was confronted by Peter. "How could you conspire to test the Spirit of the Lord?" Peter asked, and Sapphira fell at his feet and died. "This is a historical document," Marty pointed out. "It just gives you an idea of how long people have recognized that life-threatening stress can mean sudden death."

Marty explained that there is story after story indicating that intense emotion, fear, and the feeling of hopelessness can have a deleterious effect on health and become life-threatening. The stories are cataloged on Marty's computer. A seventy-nine-year-old man hears that his granddaughter has committed suicide and drops dead. A woman dies trying to save her daughter in an earthquake.

A child dies on an amusement park ride. A woman's coat is caught in an escalator in Boston and she drops dead. A driver hits a cyclist and checks on him; the cyclist is okay but

the driver drops dead. Most serious scientists dismiss anecdotal evidence. Many of these stories are referred to as "N-of-one"
stories in the medical community. "'N-of-one' means it is
based on a single case," Marty explained. Today's trend is to
demand that N equal a thousand, or ten thousand, before
anyone takes it seriously. So is the validity of an N-of-one case
dismissed by the medical establishment? I asked. "The medical community is not a monolith," Marty answered. "I take it
seriously, as do others." For him, such cases can be instructive.
"You write up one case and you learn what that one case
teaches you about an underlying biological principle."

Marty described perhaps the most famous voodoo death
case. Chang and Eng were born in May 1811, in a remote village sixty miles outside Bangkok, in what was then known as
Siam. They were conjoined twin brothers, and their condition
and birthplace became the basis for the term *Siamese twins*.

When the twins were in their teens, their mother leased
them to a British sea captain who exhibited them at carnivals
across the United States and Britain. The boys put on an old-
fashioned freak show for crowds of gawkers. The twins earned
a sizable cache of money in their years on the road, but eventually they tired of the touring.

They became U.S. citizens and moved to North Carolina,
where they built a spacious home and opened a store. The
two had been slaves to roaring crowds. Now they were slave
owners on a new plantation. The brothers celebrated a joint

wedding to sisters in 1843, provoking a national scandal amid claims it was bestial. To the astonishment of the public, their wives bore them a total of twenty-one children.

Chang and Eng lived for sixty-three years in their attached condition. One night, Chang died. "Eng awakened the next day," Marty recounted, "still attached to his dead brother. Eng announced to a nephew, 'Your uncle Chang just died, so I have to die.'" He did just that. The twins were autopsied in Philadelphia. Marty said, "The autopsy confirmed Eng's fear caused the adrenaline storm that killed him." I just stared wide-eyed.

Even in more conventional relationships, the emotional reaction to a death in the family can be traumatic, and often the "bereavement effect" kicks in—a serious physical condition. When an individual loses someone close, the survivor's feelings of loss and loneliness sometimes lead to hopelessness. Living without hope can increase the risk of damage to internal organs, including the brain.

"After a major loss, the death of a spouse or child, up to a third of the people most directly affected will suffer detrimental effects on their physical or mental health, or both," according to the *BMJ*, the *British Medical Journal*. "Such bereavements increase the risk of death from heart disease and suicide as well as causing or contributing to a variety of psychosomatic and psychiatric disorders."

Two days after Christmas 2016, actress and writer Carrie

Fisher died from multiple causes, suffered on a plane from London to Los Angeles. Twenty-four hours later, her mother, actress Debbie Reynolds, died from a stroke. Nothing in life can be crueler than the loss of a child. "It creates an overflow of stress hormones, and the heart can't take it," said Dr. Suzanne Steinbaum, director of women's heart health at Lenox Hill Hospital in New York. Dr. Anne Curtis, chair of medicine at the Jacobs School of Medicine at the University of Buffalo, told a *New York Times* reporter, "I've seen estimates that about one percent of perceived heart attacks are because of broken-heart syndrome . . . I think every cardiologist has seen cases."

Trauma of any kind can threaten lives. Marty described a study undertaken in the days following September 11, 2001. Immediately after the attack, doctors at St. Luke's–Roosevelt Hospital began compiling data on two hundred patients who had been implanted with monitors and defibrillators. These devices monitor heart rhythms. Doctors found the rate of life-threatening heart rhythms had more than doubled in patients during the month after 9/11 compared to the rate the month before.

A traumatic event more than five thousand miles away occurred on January 18, 1991, when Iraqi Scud missiles slammed into Israel. The BBC reported the incident on its website: "Iraq has attacked two Israeli cities with Scud missiles, prompting fears that Israel may be drawn into the Gulf War. Israel's largest city, Tel Aviv, and Haifa, its main seaport, were hit in the attacks, which began at 0300 local time, (0100 GMT), when most residents were asleep."

According to Dr. Samuels, a study of mortality records from the first day of the attacks found a 58 percent increase in the country's death rate over the previous day and an 80 percent increase in the death rate in Tel Aviv and Haifa, the main targets. Nobody had been hit by the missiles that day.

One of the study's authors said the analysis of hospital and morgue records reinforced the idea that some people may have been literally frightened to death. "This is the opposite of being hopeful and calm," Marty explained. "This is being hopeless and frightened."

Our brains are the neuro-hubs of our bodies, with spokes flaring to connect to every organ and system. The organs, our hearts and kidneys and all the rest, exist in the shadow of the brain. So what we think or feel has a direct effect on these organs. According to the American Psychological Association, "When muscles are taut and tense for long periods of time, this may trigger other reactions of the body." Such as death.

Marty continued, "People who are in a state without hope are like an animal in the wild trying to escape from jaguars. For each of those attacks, there is damage done to the visceral organs. And it's cumulative." That means people who live in a state of hopelessness for extended periods may be putting their bodies under long-term physiological stress.

I had been focusing on hope rather than hopelessness. Now I see it both ways. These stories and studies offered clarity. There is no antidote to hopelessness, nor is there a formula for preventing massive quantities of adrenaline from being released. Increasingly, I recognize that people who suffer from serious illnesses must find a way to hope, if only as a survival mechanism.

Physicians have a critical role to play in this effort. In my years dealing with diseases, I have crossed paths with some of the best and brightest in academic medicine. Too frequently, offering hope does not seem to be on their radar screens. They can quash hope, as my first neurologist did when he offered my MS diagnosis by telephone and basically told me to give up. The human touch is in short supply in a medical establishment overtaken by managed care and high-tech treatments. Hope is far less expensive and may be just as effective.

I asked Marty about the most important lesson he learned in his many years treating the sick. Marty said, "My main job is to give people hope. I have helped way more people, by an order of magnitude, with my words . . . than I have with any drug or medication. I think drugs and technologies are greatly overrated."

Dr. Jerome Groopman has arrived in the same place. In an address to a medical group in Southern California, Dr. Groopman, author of *The Anatomy of Hope*, discussed his own journey to understanding the need to offer hope to his patients. "I was walking back from the ward to my laboratory, after seeing people with blood diseases and cancer and AIDS. I asked myself what more I could offer these patients whom I had seen that day? The answer that came to my mind was hope. And that answer was at once both exhilarating and terrifying."

In his book, Groopman wrote, "Researchers are learning that a change in mind-set has the power to alter neurochemistry. Belief and expectation—the key elements of hope—can block pain . . . Hope can also have important effects on fundamental physiological processes like respiration, circulation, and motor function."

The mind is a powerful instrument, and hope can become self-fulfilling. What one hopes must be measured and plausible. Hoping my illnesses will disappear will not make that happen. Hope that someday soon, some new treatment will mitigate the crippling course of the disease makes sense. Maybe.

I only hope I can find the courage to take reasonable risks. I have started down that road already. I want to live my life with less anger and more grace. I cannot control my fate, but the coping choices I make are well within my power. Control? Control is fleeting. We control very little in our complicated lives. I am not captain of my ship, only a member of the crew, struggling to control the wheel.

CHAPTER 20

Anger Becomes Kid Stuff

It is not uncommon for the parents of grown children to look back across the years and wonder if we screwed up our kids. Many times the question is wistful, based on insecurity and perhaps posed after a second glass of wine. Meredith and I had our share of tough times when the children were young and illnesses showed up in our home.

Our family emerged intact from those trying years, but were we whole? Emotional damage can show itself later in life. We want to think the kids bounced back and bear no scars. They are successful and appear to be happy in their lives. We are a close-knit unit. The kids stay in touch with us and with one another. But memory hurts. Baggage that should have been put down years ago still weighs heavy. My gremlins play rough in the hours before dawn.

I asked the kids in 2017 how they would feel about coming together in a family conversation about those difficult years. I knew the thought would sound out of the blue to them, but I just wanted to hear what they would say as young adults about a time I cannot seem to forget.

The kids immediately agreed to participate, no questions asked. This was my hang-up, not theirs. Ben and Lily were visiting one Sunday in the spring. We hung out in my office at the house. I sat in my desk chair, and the kids sprawled on the floor. We got Gabe on speakerphone. Meredith joined us and we relived unhappy times. The kids demonstrated that they are in good shape, though unhappy memories can be indelible.

For Ben, the crucible always was the kitchen. "That's the space I always come back to," he told us. "I remember you guys yelling and how small that kitchen started to feel." Ben paused, scanning his memory. "I hated that room because I totally associated it with where the fights always happened."

"What do you mean?" I asked. "Fights between us?"

"Yeah," Ben answered. "You getting angry, and then Mom yelling at you. Or you yelling at somebody." Meredith jumped in. "Do you remember what the fights were about?" Ben thought for a moment. "No. I don't have very specific memories. I remember conceptually." I had no clue what Ben was talking about. I remember Meredith used to get angry with me for being too tough on the kids when things were so bad after my cancer surgeries.

Lily piped up, asking Ben if he remembered the story of my calling him a Nazi. My god, I thought. I did that? Gabe jumped in from across the country. "I remember that." I sat silently. "I remember exactly where that happened. It was at one of the houses we rented at Cape Cod. Now I know *exactly* what we're talking about." I admitted that I thought I did too.

Gabe interrupted me. "It was right outside. I remember either coming out of the house or I was still in the house and hearing Ben freaking out, saying, 'He called me a Nazi, he called me a Nazi.' I didn't understand what was going on, what that meant. But I vividly remember that." Ben was twelve then. "Yeah," Ben remarked, adding, "that was the only time you ever tried to hit me."

"I tried to hit you?" I was starting to regret proposing this conversation.

"I remember this really specifically," Ben answered. "It was the only time it ever happened. You lunged at me. I got out of the way, but you lunged at me as if you were about to smack the living crap out of me, and that's when I ran out of the house. I remember hiding behind a tree."

Beware of what you ask for. The conversation was getting out of hand. We did not hit our kids. Ever. All I could say to them at that moment was that I remembered the time frame and I was quite certain that stuff went on at a real low point for me. "What was your health at that point?" Meredith asked. It was post-cancer, and I had a stricture in my colon and I had issues, I answered. I remember being both very uncomfortable and angry. I do not say this to make excuses.

There are no excuses for terrorizing a child, only the desire to put it in context now.

I shifted the topic and brought up when I was writing the *Times* column about anger and the kids. I had treated the inquiry as a reporter just asking questions. "I remember you saying, 'Don't be afraid to tell the truth,'" Lily said. "'Don't be afraid to say whatever,' but I was really scared to say anything." Meredith asked, "Because?"

"Well, because I didn't want you to get angry again and get mad at me." Boy, I interjected. It sounds as if you guys all remember me as a monster. That did not upset me because I knew I had become a monster at times. Lily kept going. "I do remember sudden outbursts, you being angry toward yourself. It was more internal anger, like shaking your head, being like, 'This is fucking ridiculous.'" Meredith nodded her head. "That is hard to hear over and over, and I do think it was a coping mechanism, but I found it difficult to listen to."

I told the kids that I wanted to believe they had a happy childhood. Memories of those years are supposed to be uncomplicated and wonderful. Or at least just wonderful. Our lives are anything but uncomplicated. The same goes for our personalities.

"Oh, I would absolutely say we had a happy childhood," Lily said without hesitation. "I wouldn't say that I had an unhappy childhood because I can compartmentalize it," Ben added.

Poor Gabe was having trouble getting a word in from Seattle. He finally broke through the noise. "When I would hear you having an outburst, as much as it would upset and frustrate me, my natural instinct was to get away, not because I thought you were going to hurt me, but just because it was upsetting to listen to."

Meredith broached a subject that was uncomfortable for the two of us. She asked the kids, given my medical history, how much concern they had for their own health? For us, that always was the elephant in the room. Gabe and Lily both answered, "Zero."

"I don't think about it," Ben said. "I, to this day, believe that were I to have MS, it's come so far that I would have a dramatically different experience, and for that reason I was never worried about it." I looked at Ben but said not a word. "But you got an MRI, Ben," Meredith pointed out. "You were worried about it."

"I was worried about it in the sense that I started tripping and I was like, I remember the stories and I'm not stupid," Ben replied. "I have no opposition to doctors. I'm the type of person that, if I feel something, I will go to the doctor. 'Cause that's what you do." Ben was right about that.

Gabe chimed in from afar. "It certainly is always a possibility, and I know how painful it can be, but I don't think I walked away with more fear because of the family experience. I would say I would have less fear, if that makes sense." There was a momentary lull. "How can it be less?" Meredith asked. "Because you know it?"

"Yeah," Gabe answered. "We certainly had our problems, but we all walked away okay. None of us is screwed up because of it, so I feel more optimistic." Gabe sounded sure of himself. "I also don't think I live life that way, thinking, Oh, what if I got sick tomorrow? I have to imagine our experience shaped me in a more positive way that I understand if that's the worst it will be, that's not so bad."

I do not know how to assess their attitudes. There can be a fine line between circumspection and denial. But who am I to criticize when denial served me well when I was their age. Our kids observed their grandpa in the last years of his life. "I think it helped having Grandpa with MS," Lily added.

"I don't know anybody who had a grandfather playing rugby with them, you know?" Their perspective was reassuring. I asked the three of them if they thought they are better people for growing up with illness in the family. Are you more sensitive or less so? I held my breath. I could see it going either way.

"I think we all probably picked up on the ways that you can grow and become more empathetic and become more aware of the people around you at a younger age than others did," Lily answered. As an example, she pointed out, "I remember Gabe did volunteer work at Camp PALS."

I had forgotten about that. Camp PALS is a two-week

summer camp for children with Down syndrome. These kids were different from the other kids Gabe had known. They had significant physical limitations. Gabe loved working with these kids. It was a twenty-four-hour-a-day job for those weeks.

Meredith and I see that empathy in many of the news stories Gabe covers in Seattle, highly personal pieces about sick kids and the elderly. Frequently, he tells stories of struggle and has won awards for doing so. Gabe has found a niche. Ben finished business school and lives in San Francisco, doing venture capital. Lily works in Santa Monica, California, for Tastemade, a community of food and travel lovers. Though they no longer are under our roof, they are loving friends to us.

Our kids are baked and out of the oven. I love them—and equally important, I like them. They are good people. Simple satisfaction is its own reward. We done good. These young people know that nothing in life comes free. They are winning, because they are authentic. And the important question is simple: Are they happy? I am taking yes for an answer.

Epilogue: Pursuing Possibility

I am learning. Dancing with disease is a dangerous pastime. Hard lessons come with unpredictable choreography. Taking part in a groundbreaking clinical trial, on whatever terms, is a defining life experience. I know more about medical research and even about myself than I could have imagined. I have patiently endured years of ineffective therapies that might as well have been placebos. I have become inured to shattered expectations. I have to admit, I have often been negative about my future.

I am quick to dismiss possibility. Too quick. I have often expressed contempt for the very idea of hope. It never worked for me, though I hardly gave it a try. I have become a super rationalist. I insist on basing opinions and expectations solely on cold reason, discounting any emotional input. That cut out an entire dimension of life. I am not suggesting becoming a mystic or an instant believer, only a human being who occasionally opens his mind.

Then came the clinical trial. Everyone around me was breathing hope. As with any contagion, hope filled my lungs and traveled north of the neck. I ignored the feeling for a while. Then I decided to sample the stuff. I was not a convert, only a careful consumer, trying on something new and deciding if it fit. The jury is still out.

In the early stages of my involvement with Dr. Sadiq, I slowly learned a lot about the science of stem cell therapy and began writing about the MS clinical trial on my *Journey Man* blog. I wanted to share what little I knew. I described the treatment protocol I still was learning. I felt I was helping others who wanted to know more about this incredible new therapy. I posted various videos of the hideous-looking procedures Meredith and Gabe had recorded as I prepared for the future. Actually, those medical moments were not as horrible as they appeared in the videos.

The video of the stem cell infusion itself deserved an Oscar nomination. Meredith did the camera work and starred with Sadiq, keeping up a back-and-forth conversation and effectively narrating the infusion. Meredith had done her homework, and Sadiq clearly relished being provocative.

I heard from other MS patients who noted how at ease we seemed. Others who live with different diseases approached me. The sick stay on top of medical advances, watching, waiting, and wondering when their turn will come. There were expressions of thanks, literally from around the world. "Thanks, mate," came from a man in Australia. I never had been called "mate" before. Many wanted to know if they could be helped by the treatment. I had no clue and told them so.

Patients came up to me in Sadiq's waiting room, wanting to know how I was doing. Was I feeling okay? Did I see changes in my walking? I told them this was like watching grass grow. Others were gracious, and they seemed to understand stem cell therapy is no longer just science fiction.

It was clear that many patients viewed the stem cell experiment as our shared future. I was not part of the official trial, of course, and statistically I was irrelevant. That continued to niggle at me, though I doubt other patients would have cared. They knew any treatment that could help me today might serve them tomorrow.

The clinical trial was a sparkling success. The study offered struggling patients a reason to hope. Dr. Sadiq took me through the findings in late 2016.

The primary purpose of a phase-one clinical trial is to determine the safety of a drug or device. No patient appeared to have been harmed medically, so the FDA labeled the procedure as safe and tolerable. This was an important hurdle to clear, but it was the clinical results, the measurable improvements, that became the headlines for patients. Word traveled fast.

Twenty patients whose lives had been seriously compromised by their MS were included in the study. Ten were in wheelchairs; ten were not. Sadiq and I sat in his private office, going over the results of the trial. He was visibly excited by the outcome.

"Eight out of twenty patients had a functional change," he said, meaning that they could perform some of life's little tasks for the first time in memory. "Fifteen out of twenty had improvement in muscle strength." Clinical trials with less dramatic outcomes are generally judged to be successful. These numbers were promising, even inspiring.

Some patients who had been using a cane could now walk without it. Some who were using a device to help them walk didn't have to use it anymore. A few patients who had been leaning on a walker were down to only one cane. Patients who had moved with a limp now enjoyed a steadier walk. He was visibly excited about the results. It would be tough to evaluate them and not feel hope.

The Food and Drug Administration approved a phase-two trial. That is big. A phase-two trial involves a much larger patient sample and is vastly more expensive. Sadiq needed more research space to keep going. The Tisch center already has raised more than four million dollars for an expanded laboratory on a different floor. Sadiq told me that phase two will start in January 2018.

Patients pressed me to share my experience. My personal results were ambiguous and somewhat deflating. I do appear to stand straighter, and my walking is somewhat stronger.

There is nothing more to take to the bank. Dr. Sadiq believes the pulmonary embolism and diagnosis of a virulent form of psoriasis, both shortly after the first stem cell infusion, worked against me. "You are a work in progress," Sadiq said to me. We are going to come up with a new treatment plan. Perhaps a ticket to Lourdes, I thought.

My trial outcome certainly was not what I had hoped for, but the story is much larger than just me. Four hundred thousand MS patients in the United States had a stake in this trial. I think of the next generation of possible people with MS and consider what the trial might mean for them. And this experiment only was the beginning.

I continue to focus on Ben, Gabe, and Lily, who know too much about our family history and its three generations with MS to assume anything. They are well into their twenties and doing fine. If my kids remain healthy, I will be fine. I have been at this for a long time.

A friend asked if my lackluster trial results made me cynical. No, I replied. It's a little early to take my football and go home mad. I am determined to see the trial as the first mile of a long journey. With medical research, nothing happens in the blink of an eye. Years of being sick beat the need for immediate gratification out of me long ago.

When I began my inquiry into the importance of hope, that hope was difficult for me to touch. I had been burned by my failing body a few times too many. Now there have been sightings. They come and go according to my health. My challenge is to keep the spark of hope alive.

A flicker of flame burns bright in the dark, and that fire must be nurtured for the flame to continue throwing off light. I have come to believe that opening a mind can lead to a receptive heart. A person has to be ready for the possibility of hope.

For me, that fire is a beacon in the distance, and I scan the sky, looking for its light. As I consider the clinical trial and whatever is to come, I peer into the night with tired eyes, staring and trying not to blink. Hope fills my head and quickly vanishes. It is as if some spirit is toying with me.

Sightings come when I am vulnerable and most in need. That is when I open myself to possibility. When the door is open, however, fear and frustration slip in as well. My gremlins show up, and they play rough. The beasts lurking in my head do battle with hope every day.

My late father approached his ninetieth birthday wondering how he came to be so old. He knew there are only questions. For my dad, hope was not going to peel away the years. Nothing was going to change. My Old Man's initial run-in with MS had come when he was only twenty, and he went on to beat the odds and practice medicine for more than forty years. There is nothing gentle about the worlds of aging and crumbling health in the cycles of life. I am still trying to figure out where hope fits in.

I want to have a long-term relationship with hope. I really do. Making that intimate connection is a challenge. For many years I pushed hope aside, labeling it a crutch. In my research for *Chasing Hope*, smart people made the case for hope. They came from different places, but all had found the promised land. I decided I could use a little bit of the stuff. Perhaps I need a lot.

Americans by nature are optimists. Hope seems built-in. Even our political establishment has traditionally celebrated hope. "Never give in," the "Happy Warrior," former vice president Hubert H. Humphrey intoned, "and never give up." Those are words to live by in any context. Those who know hope do not give up.

In writing this book, I have learned hope can have a positive effect on the body and nourish the spirit. I approached many people to discuss hope, dreams, and beliefs. Many found hope an easy reach. I suspect my penchant for locating the roughest road to travel slowed me down.

For many, hope seems to come naturally. I wish them well. For others, hope is an article of faith. Not for me. I wonder and doubt. For those who find faith out of reach, the search for a different reservoir of strength takes more imagination. I am the product of a tight family. Meredith and the kids have provided another generation of support. People who love and care for one another foster hope.

For me, belief in the power of hope is linked to belief in

self. They go hand in hand. If we believe in ourselves, we may have discovered the secret to hope. Perhaps we need to invent our own version of hope. The support of family and friends, religion, and medicine can carry us forward. If we expect to go the distance, however, we need to look deep within ourselves.

And the questions do not end. For me, they never will. I know that. After more than a few years of wrestling with hope, I still want to understand the mystery, though I am not certain that will happen. Such a subjective notion can have no clear boundaries or bottom line.

In my world, hope expands and contracts according to need and the mood of the moment. Hope is and will remain a moving target. I have come to accept that, or at least I have an evolving tolerance for ambiguity. Not every need or doubt can be clarified, never mind resolved. Long ago, I relinquished my fear of the dark. I am comfortable not being able to see around the next bend.

I do continue to dream of better health. I will always hope to walk up the highest hill, whistling in the wind. I so want to see into the distance and know what lies ahead. Don't we all? I no longer rule out fantasies of adventure, though I know how unlikely they will continue to be. Hope is one small step for man, one giant leap for me.

The search for hope has been going on through the ages. According to Greek mythology, Pandora was Earth's first woman. When Pandora opened a vessel, releasing all evils into the world, the spirits escaped except for Elpis, the goddess of hope, who remained behind to comfort humanity.

Hope is a gift to us from us. For me, hope originates close to home. All of us are different. I never depend on hope to pull me through a crisis. Hope may yield little or nothing. I take care of business myself and know that action beats reaction when reaching for a better life.

For me, finding hope is a journey without end. I am committed to the trek. If hope darts in and out of sight, keep searching. It is somewhere. When you are tired of scanning the skies, just walk over to any mirror and take a hard look. Stand still and stare at yourself. Squint if necessary. Often we do not recognize what stands a few feet before us. Hope may be looking you in the eye.

ACKNOWLEDGMENTS

This book took a village. For a few years, I sat alone and thought about writing it but did nothing. I kept talking to my agent, Linda Loewenthal. Finally she lit a fire under me. Linda has a patient ear and an iron fist when it comes to writing book proposals. Together we birthed the idea for the book.

Beth Rashbaum, armed with skills as a freelance editor, helped me sharpen my vision and build a structure. Both of us are stubborn. We did not always see eye to eye, but we pulled it off. Beth was right more often than I. When Blue Rider Press bought the book, Becky Cole became my editor. I thought Becky was terrific, but Penguin Random House mysteriously discontinued Blue Rider Press, and Becky moved on.

Dutton, another PRH imprint, adopted the book, and Jill Schwartzman took over as my editor. By now, I was dizzy, but Jill was a calming force. She brought the manuscript in for a safe landing. Jill's enthusiasm for the book was clear. All these editors made collaboration a pleasure.

ACKNOWLEDGMENTS

Toby Wertheim, my friend and former colleague, was at my side for the duration. Toby was the chief researcher on the *CBS Evening News* with Walter Cronkite and Dan Rather. She resurrected that role and provided invaluable assistance filling in the blanks and functioning as a sounding board.

I enjoyed life in this village and hope all of us can work together again.

ABOUT THE AUTHOR

RICHARD M. COHEN is the author of two *New York Times* bestsellers: a memoir, *Blindsided*, detailing his struggles with MS and cancer and his controversial career in the news business; and *Strong at the Broken Places*, following the lives of five individuals living with serious chronic illnesses. His distinguished career in network news earned him numerous awards, including three Emmys and a Peabody. Cohen lives outside New York City with his wife, Meredith Vieira. They have three grown children.